Principles and Practice of Clinical Trial Design

Principles and Practice of Clinical Trial Design

Richard Chin, M.D.

Boston Academic Publishing
Boston, Massachusetts

PRINCIPLES AND PRACTICE OF CLINICAL TRIAL DESIGN

For an electronic version of this publication, please visit www.clinicaltrialist.com.

Please email any comments regarding this book to the author at richardchin@clinicaltrialist.com

ISBN 0-9772302-2-8

Preface

This is a book for practitioners of Clinical Research Medicine. Clinical Research Medicine is a relatively young branch of medicine, concerned with methodological issues in clinical study design, conduct, and interpretation. It is currently the primary method for establishing causal relationships between interventions and clinical outcomes in medicine. The practitioners of this field include pharmaceutical and biopharmaceutical researchers in industry, academia, and government institutions.

It is the first volume of an intended series of three. This volume focuses on design of clinical research, including topics such as patient selection, dosing, and endpoints. The primary goal of this book is to review the theoretical underpinnings of clinical trial design. The second volume will address practical aspects of conducting clinical trials, and the third will address interpretation and analysis of clinical trial results.

Table of Contents

Chapter 1: Overview of Clinical Research Medicine

1 Overview

1.1 Definition of Clinical Research Medicine

Clinical Research Medicine (CRM) is the science of designing, conducting, and interpreting clinical trials. Its goal is to understand and improve the methods for determining whether an intervention, such as a drug, a device, or a procedure, improves clinical outcome in patients. For example, it might address a question such as, "How can one determine whether or not angiotensin converting enzyme inhibitors slow the progression of renal disease?" Or it might answer a question such as, "How can one determine whether or not patients with angina benefit from coronary artery bypass surgery?" CRM is a broad field that addresses issues such as types of patients to enroll in a trial, the appropriate size of a trial, and ways of maximizing the amount and quality of information from a trial.

CRM is a branch of medicine, but it is an atypical branch, in that its primary purpose is to add to the body of medical knowledge. Most branches of medicine are concerned directly with diagnosis and treatment of patients. Surgeons operate on patients; endocrinologists manage patients with endocrine diseases; and cardiologists treat patients with cardiac problems. Physicians who practice CRM do not treat patients directly. Also, although patients enrolled in clinical trials might benefit incidentally from the drug being investigated in some instances, the goal of a clinical trial usually is not directly to benefit patients who participate in the trial but rather to discover whether a treatment is safe and/or effective.

To put it another way, a clinical trial is concerned with finding a therapy not for an individual person but rather for a group of patients with a disease. This is different from clinical practice where the goal is to treat individual patients. As an illustration, a question for a practicing clinician treating a patient not in a clinical trial may be, "Will administration of ibuprofen to Mr. X who has pain in his knee improve his symptoms?" In a clinical trial, the question may be, "Will administering ibuprofen to patients with arthritis decrease their symptoms?" It is not sufficient that ibuprofen improves knee pain in Mr. X;

the goal of a clinical trial is whether as a group, most (or sufficient proportion) of patients with knee pain of a certain type benefit. Clinical trials can eventually lead to improved therapies for a large group of patients if the treatment is demonstrated to be effective. The job of a clinical research physician is to devise the best way to design and implement such trials.

Clinical Research Medicine in Context

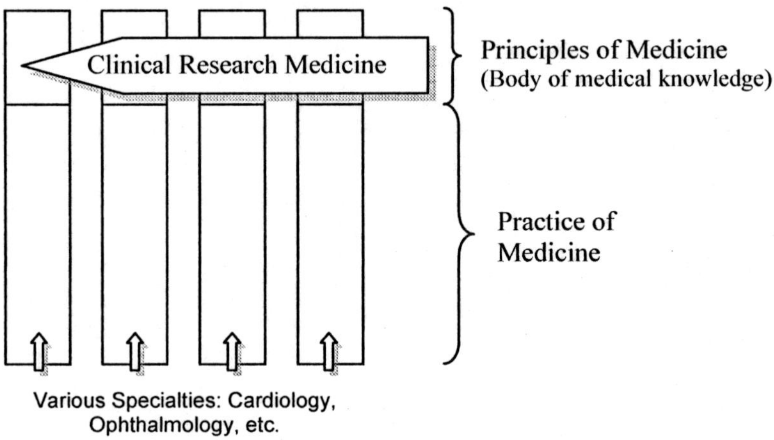

CRM is primarily a methodological science, in that it is primarily concerned with *how* to best answer such questions, not *what* the specific answer is. In other words, CRM is concerned not with what the answer is to a question such as, "Do angiotensin converting enzyme inhibitors slow the progression of renal disease?" Regardless of the answer, if the study results in a definitive result then CRM has served its purpose. Nor is it concerned with which clinical questions to study or how to apply the results to specific patients. Rather, it is concerned with what is the best way to design a trial to answer such questions.

The goal of CRM is not to be able to declare, "Angiotensin converting enzyme inhibitors do slow the progression of renal disease." Its goal is to be able to say, "A double-blind, placebo-controlled study using measured creatinine as an endpoint at 6 months will answer the question, but a single arm study using calculated creatinine at 4 weeks probably will not." As an analogy, CRM is to medicine what an architect is to the house builder, or what a coach to an athlete. In this way, CRM is more similar to other methodological fields such as statistics, education, or epistemology than to most other branches of medicine.

Note: CRM as Methodological Science

The body of data generated by CRM is usually added to specific disciplines, such as cardiology, oncology, and gastroenterology. Only the methodological knowledge is added to the body of CRM knowledge. For example, the answer to the question, "does administering angiotensin converting enzyme inhibitors to patients with diabetes slow the progression of renal disease?" would enter the body of knowledge for nephrology. The answer to the question "what is the best way to determine the answers to questions of this type where the progression of disease is slow, and surrogate markers are partially validated?" would enter the body of knowledge for CRM.

1.2 Epistemology of Medicine

As was previously mentioned, Clinical Research Medicine is only one of several possible ways of generating medical knowledge. Indeed, knowledge acquired through prospective, randomized, controlled clinical trials, which are the hallmarks of CRM, is the exception rather than the rule. Historically–even today–much of the body of medical knowledge is based on evidence other than, such as personal experience, historical knowledge, case reports, and observational studies. Commonly, intuition and pathophysiological rationale have also played important roles in shaping medical lore. Habits and practice patterns based on informal knowledge were handed down from one

Sources of Medical Knowledge

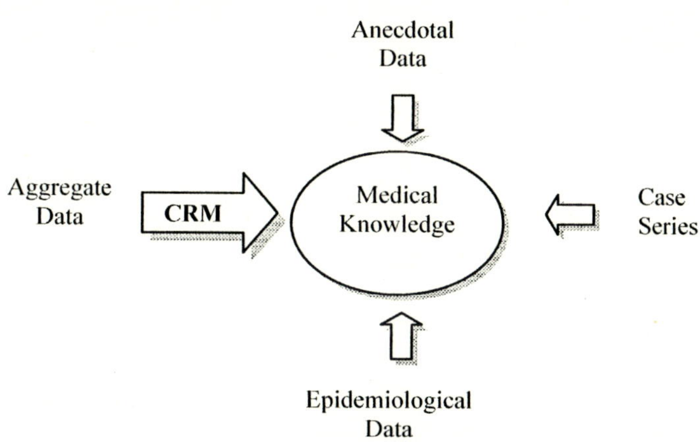

generation of physicians to the next, usually without formal verification or validation.

In many instances, the traditional methods worked adequately, and even now, clinical trials are not always necessary. For much of medicine, particularly those parts concerned with diagnosis, prognosis, education, and monitoring, traditional sources of knowledge are acceptable. Even for interventions, CRM is not always the most rigorous nor the most practical way of generating data. In cases where it is impossible to blind the treatments, in cases where it would be unethical to randomize patients, and in cases where there are extremely few patients with the disease, formal, rigorous clinical trials may not be the best option. As an example, for advance colon cancer, where the survival is <5% at 5 years, a drug that achieves 100% survival at 10 years can be proven to be efficacious without a controlled clinical trial: a small case series may be sufficient to establish efficacy.

Evidence-Based Medicine

It is often thought that "evidence based medicine" is a modern development. When this term is used, it is often with the implication physicians in the past practiced medicine without relying on evidence. Strictly speaking, this implication is inaccurate. Our forbearers in medicine practiced a form of evidence-based medicine, but the sources of evidence were of a different type. They did not have the luxury of basing their decisions on aggregate data from large trials–they had little access to such data. They relied on anecdotal data and small cases series.

The new paradigm–that of modern evidence based medicine–is different mostly in that it asserts a hierarchy of evidence, placing randomized controlled clinical trials at the top and others below that. This hierarchy is appropriate in most instances since in most cases, data generated from randomized, prospective clinical trials is more robust than anecdotal data. It is however not always appropriate, as will be discussed.

Clinical trials are expensive, difficult to conduct, and suffer from some significant validity flaws. It is neither practical nor prudent to conduct clinical trials for every therapy, and knowledge generated from other methods is both necessary and helpful in many instances. However, for many diseases, clinical trials are often the most reliable tool for establishing a causal relationship between intervention and outcome, establishing effectiveness of new therapies, and developing new treatments. This is because of the randomization, prospective treatment assignment, and large aggregate data sets that characterize well-designed clinical trials.

Unlike anecdotal data or small case series, where patient histories can be individually studied and understood, clinical trials have too many patients to allow analysis on an individual level. Rather, they require that aggregate data be analyzed. Analysis of aggregate data is neither easy nor intuitive, and fraught with cognitive illusions and intellectual fallacies. In order to avoid inaccurate or spurious conclusions, clinical trials must be designed, executed, and analyzed in a rigorous way. CRM provides the tools to accomplish this.

	CRM	Anecdotal Data	Case Series	Epidemiology
Prospective?	Yes	Yes	Sometimes	Sometimes
Active Intervention of Therapy?	Yes	Yes	No	No
Randomized, unbiased intervention?	Yes	No	N/A	N/A
Aggregate Data?	Yes	No	Sometimes	Yes
Blinded?	Yes	No	No	No
Replicate Clinical Practice?	No	Yes	Yes	Yes
Unbiased Sample?	No	No	Sometimes	Sometimes

1.3 Case Studies, Personal Observations, and Case Series

As noted above, most medical knowledge has historically been generated by accumulation of anecdotal knowledge by individual physicians and other healthcare professionals over time, passed down through generations. Informal sources of knowledge, such as personal experience, historical knowledge, published case studies and case series are effective ways of accumulating, clarifying and disseminating such knowledge. In many instances, this type of knowledge is invaluable, and has been critical in the advancement of medical care. Some examples include case series of Wegener's disease or retrospective analysis of Reye's syndrome. In addition, the intellectual tools required to observe, describe, and assimilate such knowledge usually come readily to an average physician who has been trained in the art of physical examination and diagnosis, because they draw upon similar skill sets.

The drawback to this approach is that the number of cases any individual physician or even an institution encounters is usually small. It is difficult to enlarge the data set by pooling experience of multiple physicians. Data collected by different persons, under different conditions, documented in different ways, can be difficult to collate and interpret. In addition, knowledge obtained this way is commonly fraught with confounding factors. In short, the probability of inaccurate conclusions based on these sources of knowledge tends to be higher than from randomized centralized controlled clinical trials.

Many treatments that were supported by conventional wisdom, and many practices based on knowledge distilled from thousands of physician-years of expert experience have subsequently been demonstrated to be erroneous when subjected to rigorous randomized clinical trials. A classic example is the digoxin for cardioversion. Digoxin had previously enjoyed general acceptance as being efficacious for cardioversion of atrial fibrillation until it was proven to be inert in rigorous randomized trials.

1.4 Epidemiology and Observational Data

One formal—as opposed to anecdotal—source of knowledge is epidemiology. This discipline relies on surveys, close recording of aggregate data, retrospective studies, registries, and prospective nonrandomized studies. Unlike case histories, epidemiology relies on a quantitative data set that has been collected in a consistent enough manner to allow mathematical and statistical analysis.

Example: Matches and Lung Cancer

Correlation is not causation. A classic example is the correlation divorced from causation is that between matches and lung cancer. There is a strong correlation between likelihood of someone carrying matches and probability of his or her contracting lung cancer, but matches do not directly cause cancer. Rather, many people who carry matches do so because they smoke, and smoking causes lung cancer. A randomized trial that assign one group to carrying matches and another to not carrying matches would find that there was no difference in lung cancer rates even after many years.

Epidemiology is a sister discipline of CRM. The two disciplines are similar to each other in many ways, particularly with respect to the inferential method of drawing conclusions. However, epidemiology, unlike clinical trials, does not involve an active intervention and therefore does not normally lead to causal inferences. It can establish correlations between patient characteristics or therapies and outcome, but correlations do not establish causation in and of themselves.

Formal observational knowledge can come from cross-sectional surveys, case controlled studies, and cohort studies. A cross-sectional study is a survey that collects risk factors and outcome data in a group at one point in time and examines the data for correlations. Case control study compares a group of patients with a disease and a group without the disease, to examine risk factors in the past. Cohort study examines a group with a risk factor and one without and follows them prospectively for the disease.

Note: Epidemiology and Safety Data

As an aside, one aspect of clinical research medicine that overlaps with epidemiology is the monitoring and analysis of safety data. The safety monitoring aspect of clinical research medicine relies heavily on epidemiology, and will be discussed in a later section of this book.

2 Rationale for Clinical Trials

4.1 Scientific

As noted above, there are multiple paths to medical knowledge. Reliable medical knowledge, particularly about efficaciousness of interventions, is difficult though to glean for most diseases and most interventions. There are several reasons for this, and modern randomized, controlled, prospective clinical trial can often address most of the reasons.

The first reason is that it is usually difficult to distinguish whether an outcome represents a true signal or just background noise. For example, administering a new compound to one patient (or even to 10) and observing that the patient recovers from pneumonia doesn't demonstrate that the drug cured the infection. This is because most diseases have variable outcome; anecdotal evidence are subject to tremendous biases and confounding factors; and most drugs only work partially. The patient could have spontaneously recovered from pneumonia, as many patients do.

There is tremendous variability in the onset, course, and outcome of many common diseases. Only a few of the patients who are exposed to leprosy bacteria contract the disease; only a fraction of the patients who harbor *H. pylori* develop ulcers; and only some of the patients who experience an myocardial infarction develop lethal arrhythmias. There is also great variability in response to many therapies. Statins prevent cardiovascular events in only a fraction of patients who receive them; infliximab induces a response on only in a fraction of rheumatoid arthritis patients; and aspirin relieves headache in only some patients, some of the time.

As another example, psoriasis is a disease with a waxing and waning course. Most drugs for the disease work in some patients but only sporadically, and in other patients never. Small uncontrolled series or trials in psoriasis often will yield misleading results because some drugs will seem to work when in fact it has no effect just by chance, since some patients' symptoms spontaneously regress.

Clinical trials, with (usually) large aggregate numbers, randomization, and blinding, can often overcome these issues of variability and noise.

The second reason for why medical knowledge is difficult to glean from informal observations or nonrandomized studies is that it is often difficult to determine whether a result is due to a bias or due to a real effect. For example, when a patient and/or the treating physician know that a therapy is being administered, there may be a placebo effect. For example, a physician conducting a psoriasis trial might underreport the area of body affected by psoriasis when he or she is measuring the response to the drug or placebo.

Another potential bias is imbalance between the treatment groups. The group receiving the intervention, for example, may be younger and healthier than the one not receiving it. The outcome in that group may be better than the control group, but not because of the intervention but because they were healthier to begin with. In addition, there can be regression to the mean in waxing and waning diseases, in that any therapy administered during flares will seem to improve symptoms in some patients, just due to the natural history of the disease.

Clinical trials can ameliorate some of these biases and issues. Blinding can reduce the placebo effect and randomization can reduce imbalances in patient characteristics between the groups.

The third argument against informal observations as the sole source of medical knowledge is that given any set of data, and given sufficient numbers of analysis of subgroups and endpoints, it is possible to link almost any therapeutic intervention to an outcome. In other words, if the data is analyzed enough times in enough different ways, one can often find a convincing association between therapy and outcome. On average, looking at the data in 20 different ways can be expected to yield one spurious association with a p value of 0.05 or less.

Prospective clinical trials prespecify one primary endpoint. This minimizes the risk of spurious results. By convention, a randomized, prospective clinical trial that demonstrates a difference between a treated group and an untreated group for the prespecified primary endpoint with a p value of less than 0.05 is accepted as having established a causal relationship. This convention does not eliminate the possibility of spurious results, but does make it much less likely, and establishes a common language and common ground for decisions on whether an intervention was effective.

The fourth and the most important reason against informal knowledge, especially knowledge based on retrospective data, is that although in some special cases, it is possible to establish causation—i.e., that a drug can treat or cure a disease—based on purely anecdotal or informal knowledge, in most cases, it is not possible to establish causation without randomized intervention. For example, patients who ingest aspirin might be found to have low incidence of cardiovascular risk. Based on that information alone, it is possible that aspirin lowers the risk of cardiovascular events, but other possible reasons cannot be ruled out. An alternate reason might be that patients who exercise more tend to injure their knees more and tend to take aspirin for their aching joints. Or, it may be that a diet low in fat is more likely to cause dental caries and patients therefore take more aspirin to relieve the dental pain.

The opposite is also true: confounding may mask causal association. As an example, patients who appear to be sicker might be more likely to receive thrombolytics than one who does not. The patient populations would then be different between those who received and did not receive the thrombolytics, and the group receiving the intervention may not do better than the one receiving it. It is possible with multivariate analysis to tease out some of the effects of the differences in the patient population, but this has significant limitations, not the least of which is that the multivariate modeling can only adjust for measured confounders.

Therefore, clinical trial—ideally, randomized prospective clinical trial—is the optimal (or sometimes the only) way of establishing clear causation. In a randomized prospective trial, the choice of treatment that a patient received is arbitrary and uninfluenced by preferences or characteristics of the patient and the physician. And the intervention precedes the measured clinical outcome. Only by randomizing patients to intervention versus non-intervention/ placebo in a prospective fashion, with the intervention clearly being assigned independent of patient or physician characteristics and occurring prior to measurement of the outcome, can causation be definitely established.

In sum, the advantages of a rigorous, randomized, well-controlled clinical trial is that it can establish causation, limit the placebo effect, avoid spurious conclusions, and yield reliable information.

4.2 Regulatory

The second major reason for performing randomized clinical trials is that new drugs and therapies must demonstrate efficacy in such a trial before it can be registered. This is related to the scientific reason, in that the scientific rationale drives the regulatory requirements. Regulatory approvals of new therapies generally require clear evidence of efficacy and safety that usually can come only from well designed and conducted randomized prospective clinical trials.

3 Limitations of Clinical Trials

Although clinical trials, in many ways, are the gold standard for investigating interventions, they are imperfect, and have important limitations. The two most critical limitations are generalizability and effectiveness. In addition, there are several less critical, though still important, limitations regarding some fundamental assumptions behind clinical trials and analysis of aggregate biological data. These assumptions are sometimes not appropriate. Furthermore, data from clinical trials can be only a part of the considerations that go into a medical decision and care of patients.

Generalizability refers to the appropriateness of extrapolating the results of the study to the general patient population as a whole. Clinical trials normally enroll a sample or a subset of patients with a disease, not everyone who has the disease. For example, there might be millions of patients with multiple sclerosis worldwide, but a clinical trial might enroll only a thousand of the patients. The data from the thousand patients might be used to guide treatment of all other multiple sclerosis patients. This is appropriate only if the results of the study are generalizable.

In order for a clinical trial to be truly generalizable, it ought to enroll a random sample of patients with a disease, the patient population should reflect the patient population at large, and it should manage the patients in a way similar to the way they would be managed by a typical physician in clinical practice. Otherwise, the likelihood that the overall patient population will respond to the intervention in the same way as the patients in the clinical trial is diminished.

None of these conditions are fully fulfilled in a typical clinical trial. Enrollment is never at random, inclusion and exclusion criteria often define a patient population somewhat different from the patient population at large, and the patients in a clinical trial receive different type of care than the patient population at large.

Closely related to generalizability is effectiveness. Clinical trials test efficacy, not effectiveness, of a drug. The goal of a clinical trial is usually to determine the true difference between a drug and placebo. In order to accomplish this goal, many artificial restrictions and atypical processes are common in clinical trials. This includes frequent visits to the physician, extra attention by the health care staff, processes to maximize compliance, prohibition of concomitant medications, and so on.

Not uncommonly, the results of clinical trial may overestimate or underestimate the effect likely to be seen in real life. For example, overestimation may occur since compliance tends to be higher in well-run clinical trials. On the other hand, clinical trial results are often analyzed using rigorous analysis often imputing worst possible outcome against the drug arm for missing data, and therefore conclusions may underestimate the effectiveness of the drug.

The question of how much clinical benefit a drug will deliver in community clinical practice is a different question from whether the drug can improve outcome in a tightly controlled clinical trial. Sometimes called external validity, effectiveness is influenced factors such as compliance in real life, interaction with other medications, benefit from placebo effect, etc.

In addition to the above two limitations, there are some assumptions and approximations that are implicit in clinical trials including assumption of linearity of biological phenomena, assumption of a normal distribution for numerous aspects of patient and outcome parameters, assumption that environmental factors (e.g., bacterial resistance patterns) and clinical practice patterns remain stable over time, and so on. These assumptions are usually reasonable but never completely true. Assumption of linearity of blood pressure, for example, is necessary in order for mean blood pressure to be calculable. The difference between 95 mmHg and 100 mmHg (of 5 mmHg) is assumed to be equivalent to the difference between 120 mmHg and 125 mmHg. Otherwise, adding and subtracting blood pressure to derive mean blood pressure would be meaningless. An assumption that practice patterns and patient characteristics remain constant from the first patient to the last patient is required in order to aggregate clinical trial data for analysis in a meaningful way.

In some cases, these assumptions are clearly inappropriate. For example, leprosy rates have decreased over time, *H. pylori* is nearing extinction in some populations, and asthma rates are increasing rapidly in industrialized countries. And practice patterns and patients certainly change over time. If a trial lasts for a long time, the consistency of patient and clinical treatment characteristic over time cannot be guaranteed.

Also, there are inherent assumptions about definition of diseases and patient groups. For example, all trials must define inclusion and exclusion criteria that rely on assumptions about whether and which patients can be grouped together – whether to distinguish for example between patients with different genotypes or from different geographies. The assumptions about the group of patient enrolled, that they share similar pathophysiology and response to therapy are usually but not always appropriate. For example, grouping patients with ST elevation myocardial infarctions (myocardial infarction's) with patients with non-ST elevation myocardial infarction's may be appropriate for a trial of bivalirudin but not for thrombolytics since thrombolytics do not appear to benefit the non-ST elevation myocardial infarction patients. Grouping patients with myocardial infarction's with patients undergoing bypass surgery may be appropriate for a trial of antiplatelet agent but not for a trial of anti-inflammatory agent.

Ideally, conducting a trial in a highly homogeneous population, or within the smallest subcategorization of patients, would yield the highest likelihood that the results can be generalizable to that population, but there is not enough resources to conduct clinical trial, with current methodologies, in each niche indication. It is not practical, for example, to do a study just on patients with anterior myocardial infarction's, with ST elevation greater than 2 mm, who have had symptoms for 4-6 hours. Instead, the category of enrollable patients might be patients with anterior or inferior myocardial infarction's, with ST elevation greater than 1 mm, who have had symptoms for 0-12 hours.

Another limitation is the practical limitation on the amount of data that can be collected. Given the finite number of patients that can be enrolled in a clinical trial, and finite length of follow-up, it is often impossible to collect the amount of data one would like. Estimation of rare safety events can be particularly difficult, because rare events may not appear in even a large database. Also, demonstrating an effect on a rarely occurring endpoint can be difficult, and sometimes surrogates are required.

There are also some fundamental assumptions about drugs themselves that are sometimes not appropriate. For example, a common assumption is that the drug dose can be reproduced from pill to pill and batch to batch. That is, that 100 mg of a drug will always have the same exact amount of drug and consistent amount of other ingredients and contaminants. For biologics, this assumption can be particularly tenuous, and it is sometimes necessary to test the biologic that come from several different batches and have a range of characteristics such as molecular weight, N terminal modifications, and glycosylation patterns.

Similarly, there are often constraints on the way that the patients are treated with regard to dosing frequency, compliance, and other characteristics that may be in conflict with the assumptions of clinical trials. These limitations will be discussed later in this book.

Finally, much of medical treatment is driven by art rather than science. Even in instances where data regarding intervention and outcome is available, it is sometimes overshadowed by non-scientific considerations such as tradition, patient preference, and practical considerations. For example, many physicians often base medical decisions not solely on data and teleological considerations but also on deontological factors such as practice guidelines or knowledge of what his peers are doing in a particular situation – standard of care, in other words. For example, they may prescribe IV nitroglycerin to myocardial infarction patients because other physicians in the city do so, while in another city, different practice may prevail.

Often, physicians also base interventions on the philosophy that making the patients feel better through comfort, reassurance, and education is as important or more important than whether the clinical outcome is improved. Of course, patients' preferences, family and caregivers' preferences, and logistic constraints such as cost and availability of therapy (particularly in less affluent societies) also play an important role.

4 Characteristics and Performance Criteria of CRM

4.1 Characteristics of Clinical Research Medicine

As was previously noted, the goal of a clinical trial is not directly to maximize benefit to the patients in the trial but rather to discover whether a treatment is effective and safe. Viewed another way, the goal of the clinical trial is to render causal conclusions between the treatment and outcome, both efficacy outcome and safety outcome. In order to accomplish this, the trials are designed, conducted, and analyzed along specific principles, and share particular characteristics. This set of principles and characteristics make up

CRM. For example, CRM relies on statistical inference and aggregate data that are collected in a quantitative manner to render causal conclusions.

Perhaps the most salient characteristic of CRM is that it is a stochastic science: it is a probabilistic science. This is because, as was previously mentioned, unlike some other scientific fields, there is tremendous variability in the subject matter when it comes to clinical trials. Patients are heterogeneous, they may be taking different concomitant medications, practice patterns differ, and so on.

Of course, there are many branches of science where the outcome is variable and the effects of intervention are also variable. In these cases, there are several traditional approaches to elucidating cause and effect. The most common method is the reductionist one. Classical physics provides a good example. In physics, complex phenomena are broken down into basic elements, such as mass, speed, inertia, etc. and basic laws have been elucidated to describe and predict behavior of objects. In physics, if mass and velocity are known, then momentum can be calculated with certainty. Reductionist approaches are helpful when the scientific problem can be broken down into small pieces, each piece investigated separately, and then a fuller understanding achieved by reassembling the pieces. For example, each piece of a metabolic cycle might be studied in isolation and knowledge of the overall metabolic cycle built up one step at a time.

In rare cases, the variability in clinical trials can be addressed by classic reductionist methods – for example, by enrolling a very homogeneous patients population or a population that has a specific genetic marker. Perhaps some day in the future, pathogenesis of diseases and variability among patients will be understood well enough so that a reductionist approach can be generally applied to medicine. However, the current state of medical knowledge is such this is not possible. There are too many independent variables in diseases, patients, and interventions. It is not possible for example to identify all genes, all environmental factors, and other factors to predict with certainty how a patient will respond to a therapeutic intervention. (In a small number of cases, the contributing effect of one factor, such as tumor or sepsis is so overwhelming that the outcome is highly predictable but as previously mentioned, these examples are rare.)

Instead of a reductionist method, clinical trials rely on collecting aggregate data. The problem of variability is addressed via repeated measurements on multiple patients. Rather than using a reductionist approach utilizing deterministic methos, clinical trials are conducted and analyzed with statistical methods (apart from a few specific corners of CRM, such as metabolism and pharmacokinetic/pharmacodynamic).

Note: Stochsticism *vs.* Determinism

Traditional science is based on deductive reasoning: linear conclusion based on assumptions and logics. Clinical research medicine is a probabilistic science, and relies on induction and inference for conclusions (but based on strict conventions relating to standards for accepting such inferences, such as p value <0.05).

Indeed, statistical analysis on aggregate data lies at the heart of CRM. CRM is an inferential science. It is not possible to draw any conclusions from clinical trials with absolute certainty. From clinical trials, it is only possible to infer that something is likely or unlikely. This type of science, a probabilistic science, is called stochsticism, and it is very different from deductive or deterministic science.

In general, a clinical trial is concerned with testing a hypothesis, generally with the requirement that the results have less than 5% likelihood of occurring by chance if the null hypothesis were true. Its goal is to determine whether an intervention has an effect on outcome.

However, a clinical trial is sometimes concerned with determining the mechanism of action, such as will a non steroidal anti-inflammatory drug (NSAID) improve arthritis, and sometimes it is concerned with diagnostics, such as will response to ibuprofen predict the likelihood of responding to other NSAID or the likelihood of worsening symptoms over the next 5 years, etc. But these tend to be the exceptions rather than the rule. CRM is an applied science, not basic science, and the goal to discover actionable knowledge that can be used by clinicians.

Also, a clinical trial is a scientific experiment and like other scientific experiments, the goal is to keep all variables constant except for one–in this case the intervention–and to measure whether there is a difference in outcome between the group that received the intervention and the one that did not. For example, in a trial of a new drug for knee pain, it would not be prudent to have some patients receive acetaminophen and some not, to have some patients rest their knee and others run marathons, put all the acute knee pain in one treatment group and chronic in the other, etc. While there are various techniques to compensate for imbalances, such as matching, multivariate analysis, etc., the most effective way to minimize imbalance between the treatment groups is through prospective randomization.

A clinical trial assigns patients prospectively to a treatment group. Usually, the assignment is via randomization. This is necessary in order to establish causation. This is in contrast to an observational study where the physician or patient selects the treatment. It prescribes an intervention.

A clinical trial assesses outcome with a quantitative measurement that can be applied across many patients by many assessors. This is in contrast to qualitative assessments or assessments that are so highly operator dependent as to make aggregation of data meaningless.

A clinical trial also involves people. As such, there are strict constraints on how a trial is conducted. For example, Phase I trials are usually conducted in a dose escalation manner. Nonparallel dosing groups violates a cardinal rule in clinical trial design, but parallel dosing is not possible in most first-in-man trials because of patient safety issues, which obviously trump all other considerations.

Example: A Typical Clinical Trial

Let's trace the steps in experimental design that leads from a non-causal associative knowledge to well controlled prospective randomized trial. As an example, let's discuss how one might investigate the question, "what should Mr. X do when he has an episode of knee pain?" The first step might be to review things in the past that might have helped his pain, such as hot bathes, ibuprofen, massages, etc. In this way, we might establish a correlation between improvement in pain and an intervention, but it is almost impossible to establish causation. For example, there might be a good correlation between massages and relief of pain, but it may be that Mr. X received massages only when the pain lasted more than a week, and it just happened that the maximum duration of this particular type of pain was no more than 10 days.

The simplest example of a prospective clinical trial might be to give Mr. X some randomimab the next time he has knee pain, and to determine whether the pain improves. This is a clinical trial in it most simplest form – an unblinded, uncontrolled, nonrandomized, prospective clinical trial.

In order to do this, though, it would be necessary to define what improvement means, and how to measure the improvement—is it sufficient if Mr.X feels better, or would objective signs such as swelling need to improve?

Also, it is not possible to determine from one experiment whether randomimab was the cause of his relief. It might have been a fluke.

So one might try giving Mr. X randomimab for his knee on several occasions when he has knee pain. This would prove reproducibility, but then the next question would be whether the natural history of his knee pain was such that it would spontaneously improve on its own.

The next refinement of the clinical trial might be to alternate or use some random sequence or treatment. He might receive randomimab on some occasions and nothing on others. If there were a correlation between randomimab and relief, this would be stronger evidence. The next question then becomes whether there is placebo effect.

A better method might be to alternate randomimab with placebo. This would help establish a causal relationship between randomimab and relief, if one were to assume certain things, such as: the knee pain is same type of pain in each occurrence, the patient remained blinded, etc. By causal relationship, I mean the conclusion that if Mr.X were to receive randomimab for his knee pain in the future, then his pain would improve.

These sets of experiments however, would not necessarily lead to the conclusion that if other patients with knee pain were to receive randomimab then they would improve as well. In order to establish that, a group of patients with knee pain would need to be tested. Also, in many diseases, such as stroke, it is not possible to repeat multiple trials of a medicine on the same patient because the patient does not return to baseline, or only has one or few episodes of the symptoms in his or her life. Because of these and other reasons, clinical trials ' are generally conducted in a group of patients with a disease. It is of course Important to define which disease population of patients to test. Fortunately, often, clinical practitioners have defined groups of patients into "diseases" and it is often useful o use these categories. However, these should just be a starting point.

4.2 The Practice of CRM

Although CRM is largely a methodological discipline, it has important practical aspects. It is methodological in that like the field of statistics, CRM is largely concerned with the theoretical issues, such as what kind of data to collect, in what fashion, and what kind of conclusions to draw from the data. It has a practical aspect in that there are logistics, real-world issues and constraints that must be addressed in order to collect and verify the data. The practice of CRM (as opposed to the principles or theory of CRM) can be divided into a clinical and a no clinical aspect.

The primary clinical aspect is protection of patient safety. In the course of a clinical trial, clinical knowledge has to be brought to bear real-time in order to assess safety events, understand them, and collate them – and in some cases alter– the conduct of the study in response to safety signals. In the design of a clinical protocol, clinical judgment is required to insure that the dose and other aspects of the trial protect patient safety.

It is because of this aspect of CRM that it is a branch of medicine, and more importantly, why the most important principle of CRM is the same as in any branch of medicine: do no harm.

After a drug is marketed, there is additional safety surveillance responsibility that is part of CRM, and in that, clinical judgment and practice is required.

The nonclinical practical aspect of CRM includes assurance of quality, GCP, and other practical aspects of running a trial and assuring data integrity.

5 Steps in Clinical Development

The detailed discussion of clinical development phases is not presented in this volume. However, they are briefly summarized below.

Preclinical Phase

The preclinical phase includes discovery, development, and toxicology phases. Discovery phase is the basic research phase where potential biological targets are studied and candidate molecules are discovered. For example, identification of HMG-CoA reductase as a potential target for cholesterol control, and development of drug candidates to block the enzyme would be performed in this phase. Activities that might occur in this phase include development of assays to screen for biological activity, screening, lead optimization such as chemical modifications to increase half life or bioavailability, formulation, testing of the candidate molecules in animal models of the disease, etc. In addition, this phase include toxicology, or basic testing in animals to insure that there is no serious untoward safety concerns with the drug.

Pilot Studies/Experimental Medicine

Pilot studies to demonstrate proof of concept are sometimes performed if good preclinical models do not exist, or if a drug is already on the market and is know to be safe. Sometimes termed proof of concept studies or experimental medicine, these studies require that the safety of the molecule be reasonably well characterized, and that there be clinical or surrogate endpoints that can yield highly predictive data. For example, such a study may be appropriate for an antibody (since antibodies in general have low toxicity) designed to treat rheumatoid arthritis

Phase I

Phase I studies are usually small (30-80 patient) first-in-man studies. They are designed to determine initial safety/tolerance profile, maximal tolerated dose, and initial pharmacokinetic/pharmacodynamic and metabolism of the drug.

Phase II

Phase II studies are usually intended to further define tolerability/safety, to select a dose and obtain some early indications of a drug's efficacy. It generally yields information to help design Phase III studies, such as accurate sample size calculations. It can also afford an opportunity to validate measurement instruments for use in Phase III.

Although in some instances, Phase II studies use same patient populations and endpoints as Phase III, this is usually the exception, and surrogate makers and enriched patient populations are often used in Phase II.

Phase III

Phase III studies are generally pivotal studies meant to demonstrate clear efficacy of a drug and to establish a safety database large enough to support a marketing application. They are hypothesis-testing studies.

Phase IV

Phase IV studies usually are postmarketing studies designed to collect further safety information on a drug. They are often uncontrolled observational studies. These studies are often the only way to characterize rare safety events and to collect effectiveness data, which is distinct from efficacy data available from Phase III.

Other Types of Trials

In addition to the above, there are numerous types of special trials, including bioequivalence studies, special population studies, vaccination studies, etc.

Chapter 2: General Issues in the Design of Clinical Trials

1 Background

1.1 Types of Clinical Trials

There are multiple ways to categorize clinical trials, but one of the most important distinctions is between descriptive trials and hypothesis-testing trials.

Descriptive trials are trials such as open label safety trials and pharmacokinetic/pharmacodynamic studies, in which the goal is to characterize a clinical or laboratory phenomena after an intervention. They do not test hypothesis and do not establish causation between intervention and clinical outcome. Nonetheless, they are often important for hypothesis generation, efficacy characterization, safety characterization, establishment of risk benefit, and guidance of therapy. Phase I studies are usually descriptive trials.

Descriptive trials can sometimes be confused with historically controlled trials, but the distinction between the two is important. Descriptive trials are not intended to establish correlation and causation. Studies that are called uncontrolled trials are often actually historical controlled, and are intended to establish causation. For example, a trial that describes the long term survival rate after administration of a chemotherapeutic agent can be descriptive if the primary endpoint of short term survival has already been established, and the long term survival is to add additional information to guide use of the drug. It may be an uncontrolled trial if its goal is to establish initial efficacy, there is good historical control data, and the anticipated benefit is far greater than historical controls—for instance, if the survival rate is 0% after 1 year and the drug is expected to result in 80% survival.

Descriptive trials are important, but at the heart of CRM are trials that test hypothesis. This is because the main goal of CRM is to determine whether an intervention improves outcome. A randomized, controlled, prospective clinical trial is usually the most definitive way to obtain this information. This book is mostly concerned with design of such trials, and methods for optimizing such trials.

Of course, most hypothesis-testing trials usually include multiple descriptive secondary endpoints that are ancillary to the primary endpoint. In a sense, almost all studies have descriptive components. Strictly speaking, it would be more correct to classify endpoints rather than trials as hypothesis-testing or descriptive. But by convention, if a study has a primary endpoint that is testing a hypothesis, the study is considered to be hypothesis-testing, and if not, descriptive. The critical difference between the descriptive and hypothesis-testing endpoints are establishment of causal relationships.

Within the category of hypothesis-testing trials, the archetypical trial is the randomized, prospective, parallel group, placebo-controlled, two-arm trials. Essentially all clinical trials are prospective, since it is otherwise almost impossible to establish causation, but the other typical characteristics of hypothesis-testing trials are variable.

Most trials are randomized because randomization is usually the most rigorous way to assign treatment. All hypothesis-testing trials assign patients to treatment in some fashion, even if it is an assignment method other than randomization. Without assignment, it is not possible to establish causation in a rigorous fashion, because this is the only way to make certain that the treatment choice has not been influenced by a factor associated with the outcome. For example, if the treatment choice is left up to the physician, he might consciously or subconsciously select the sickest patients to receive the drug and less sick to receive placebo.

Most hypothesis-testing trials are parallel group, because it is usually the cleanest way to compare groups, but several other temporal sequencing schemes exist, including dose escalation and crossover. These are discussed in a later chapter.

Clinical trials most often have two arms, and almost always test for superiority of one arm over the other. However, multiple arms are possible, and nonequivalence and noninferiority trials are possible. Nonequivalence trials are multiple dose trials where the goal is to determine whether one arm is different from the others. In noninferiority trials, the goal is to demonstrate that the two arms are relatively similar. In all cases, however, there is at least one control group.

Most trials also tend to be directed toward treating rather than preventing disease. However, there are multiple other types of trials. There are trials in patient with a disease where the goal is to reverse the disease, such as antibiotic trials in patients with pneumonia; trials in patients with a disease where the goal is to prevent worsening of the disease, such as chemotherapy in cancer patients; trials in patients at risk for a disease where the goal is to prevent the disease, such as chickenpox vaccine in young children. Even for the same disease, such as psoriasis, there can be several different potential types of trials, such as trials to induce remission or to maintain remission.

In addition, there are multiple additional degrees of freedom in clinical trial design, such as fixed dose *vs.* weight based dose *vs.* dose titrated to effect. This section addresses these and other topics.

Invariant requirement of hypothesis-testing clinical trials	**Variable properties of hypothesis-testing clinical trials**
• Prospective intervention • Assignment to treatment groups • At least one control group • Null hypothesis	• Randomization *vs.* other ways of assignment • Number of treatment groups • Superiority *vs.* other testing • Type of outcome being tested

1.2 Null Hypothesis and Standard of Proof in Clinical Trials

In addition to prospective intervention, assignment of treatment groups, and use of at least one control arm, all hypothesis-testing clinical trials share an additional invariant feature: the null hypothesis. All hypothesis-testing clinical trials are built around the null hypothesis, and therefore understanding the rationale for the null hypothesis is critical to the understanding of clinical trial design.

A priori, the most useful hypothesis to test in clinical trials would seem to be a hypothesis that posits something, such as "this intervention increases survival by 10%," or "this intervention reduces blood pressure by 10 mmHg." However, clinical trials use null hypothesis such as: "this intervention has no effect." This is a peculiarity that is fundamental to the design and science of clinical trials.

The need for the null hypothesis arises because CRM is a stochastic, or a probability-based, science and in such a science, it is not possible to prove that something is true or likely. It is only possible to prove that something is unlikely. By demonstrating that it is unlikely that the intervention has no effect, one establishes that the intervention probably does have an effect on the outcome.

In other sciences such as physics, an experiment that produces a predicted result can be considered to validate the hypothesis. This is because the results are often fully determined – in other words, a unique set of causes exists for a unique set of results (after applying Occam's Razor). For example, if matter is converted into energy, and the resultant amount of energy is known, then the amount of starting matter must be of a certain value. As an analogy, 2 x 10 is always 20 in a deterministic science, and 4 x 10 is always 40.

In clinical trials, this is not the case. Clinical trials are stochastic, and it is not possible in stochastic science to prove or disprove something definitively. One cannot even establish that an outcome is likely the result of some precedent event. One can only establish that an outcome is not likely the result of a precedent event. Because of the variability in clinical course, a completely ineffective intervention could, purely by chance, yield clinical trial results that make it appear that the intervention is effective and vice versa. In other words, 2 x 10 is usually 20 but could sometimes be 40, and 4x10 is usually 40 but could be 20 sometimes. And an intervention that decreases blood pressure by 10 mmHg would decrease blood pressure by 10 mmHg in clinical trials on average if an infinite number of trials were run, but for any given trial, it could decrease it by 9 mmHg, 15 mmHg, or even increase it.

Determinism

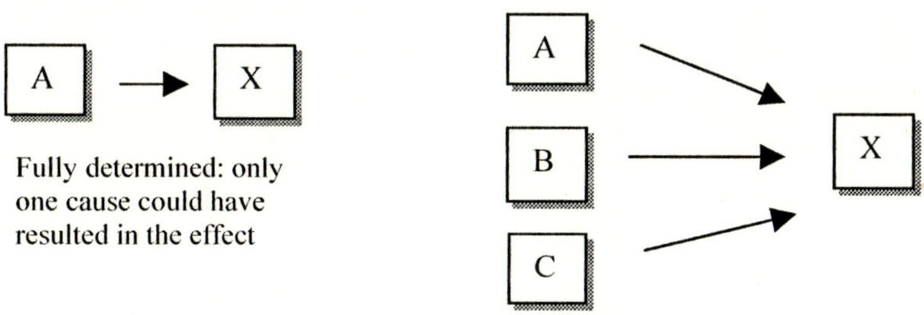

Fully determined: only one cause could have resulted in the effect

Overdetermined: many causes could have resulted in the effect

In addition, because clinical trials are stochastic, and because of the variability inherent in medicine, clinical trials results are overdetermined (my apologies to philosophers and psychoanalysts for using this word in a different sense than the original meaning). There is more than one set of circumstances that can lead to similar clinical trial results. Therefore, it is not sufficient to show merely that an outcome is a reasonable consequence of an intervention, since that doesn't exclude the possibility that the same outcome is a reasonable consequence of random chance. For example, if a trial shows that an intervention decreases blood pressure by 10 mmHg, it doesn't necessarily prove that the drug decreases blood pressure by that much. Similarly, it is not enough to show that active arm having 10% mortality and placebo arm having 20% is consistent with the drug being active. If there is enough variability in the population, the same result could also be consistent with the drug not being active – a 10 mmHg drop in blood pressure could be from placebo effect. Or the drug might really decrease blood pressure by 5 mmHg, or actually increase it but the placebo effect is overwhelming the drug effect.

Instead, the only way to establish a causal explanation is to rule out all other potential explanations.

Because of this, null hypothesis is used in clinical trials. Since it is not possible to prove that an intervention caused the outcome, one must show that lack of intervention (probably) did not cause the outcome. In order to draw a conclusion that the result was due to an intervention, one must show that it is unlikely that it was not due to intervention. This is why the null hypothesis usually is stated in the form, "there is no difference between the active and the control groups."

This approach of establishing cause and effect by disproving the null hypothesis has inherent limitations. The conventional p value of 0.05 is arbitrary. The outcome is dichotomous, and doesn't yield information such as the magnitude of the certainty or the point estimate of the effect. A trial therefore could be positive without being great enough in magnitude to be of clinical significance. It doesn't yield information about subgroups. It is a dichotomous answer to a multifaceted question. Nonetheless, it is the best method devised to date to investigate causal relationship between clinical intervention and clinical outcome.

2 Performance Criteria for Well Designed Clinical Trials

2.1 Criteria

The criteria that distinguish well designed trials from poorly designed ones are multiple. A clinical trial is a scientific endeavor, so the first criterion is:

are the results accurate? In other words, does it render an accurate answer to the hypothesis? This is sometimes referred to as internal validity.

Furthermore, it is an applied science, so the second criterion is: are the results of the study useful? Usefulness can be divided into three parts. In most cases, positive results are more useful than negative result, so is the study optimized for likelihood of positive result? However, positive results are only useful if the question that is being posed does an adequate job of capturing the manifestations of the disease – it is not useful to improve one symptom of a disease while worsening another. So, is the question being posed by the trial well formed? Also, is the study designed so that the results are applicable to real-life patients, and will they be of use to the practicing clinician? This is sometimes referred to as external validity.

A clinical trial is different from most applied sciences in that the subjects are human, so the third criterion, and a criterion that is more important than all others, is: does the trial protect patient safety and is it ethical? Does it limit risk to subjects by involving the fewest number of patients necessary? Finally, clinical trials are expensive and difficult to carry out, so the fourth criterion is: is the trial efficient and feasible to carry out? These criteria are discussed below.

2.2 Are the Results Accurate?

The most important goal of a well-designed clinical trial is to render clear and accurate answer to the hypothesis. In other words, it must yield the correct answer to the question being asked, which is usually whether the drug candidate is effective. The result of a clinical trial can be classified into three categories: accurate result, inaccurate result, and uninterpretable result.

Accurate result: A well-designed clinical trial will maximize the likelihood that a trial will yield accurate result: positive result (statistically significant) when the drug works, and negative result (lack of significance) when the drug does not. Even a well-designed trial will not guarantee an accurate result, but it will maximize the likelihood.

Inaccurate result: Statistical fluke or a fundamental design flaw(s) can lead to an inaccurate result: positive result when the drug does not actually work, and negative result when it does work.

Uninterpretable result: Worse than an inaccurate result, and unfortunately seen nearly as frequently are uninterpretable results. This can be due to insufficient data, for example because the study was underpowered, did not test a high enough dose, or was terminated too early. It may also be due to poor quality data, because of missing data, patient dropouts, unreliable measurements, etc. It may also be due to failure to minimize bias, such that the results are not reliable. All of theses flaws can lead to results being unreliable or not robust to sensitivity analysis.

There are natural imperfections in the trials. There might be too many dropouts. There are issues of imputation. There might be inadvertent unblinding. There might be regression to the mean. There might be too much interobserver variability. There might be training effects and other biases introduced by the study itself.

Also, like all scientific experiments, clinical trials are conducted in controlled setting. The patients are homogeneous; they receive regular medical attention, etc. This in itself can introduce biases. There are multiple challenges in keeping the trial free of biases, both systematic and random.

Good clinical trial design minimized the likelihood of these, and makes the analysis plan robust to the errors as much as possible. In other words, a well-designed clinical trial has internal validity: the results indicate a causal relationship between the intervention and outcome when such a relationship really exists and vice versa.

2.3 Is the Study Question Well Formed?

Is the Study Designed to Maximize Likelihood of a Positive Result?

In most instances, a safe and effective therapy is more useful to the clinician than one that is not. Therefore, demonstrating that a therapy is safe and effective for a disease is more desirable than demonstrating that it isn't, except for cases where an ineffective therapy is already in wide use. Therefore a clinical trial design should maximize the likelihood of positive study results. This is different from the question of whether the results are accurate. A study that is well designed, in addition to yielding accurate results, also poses the right question. For example, a study looking at the impact on 30-day mortality of 100 mg of a certain drug in severe sepsis patients may yield an accurate result that it has no impact. However, it may be that 200 mg of the drug in moderate sepsis patients has a beneficial impact on 60 day mortality. Selecting the right patient population, the right dose, and the right endpoint have critical impact the likelihood of success.

Does the Study Question Address the Appropriate Issues?

It is important that the question have construct validity. For instance, if the purpose of the study is to determine whether a thrombolytics has beneficial effect on myocardial infarction patients, including the incidence of re-ischemia and congestive heart failure without including death as part of a composite endpoint might lead to inappropriate conclusions. This is because congestive heart failure and re-ischemia rates might increase even when the therapy is providing a benefit. Patient who would have died might live but with congestive heart failure. Similarly, measuring myelitis without accounting for renal failure in lupus patients may yield erroneous conclusion that the drug is beneficial when in fact it shifts one manifestation of the disease to another.

Are the Results Generalizable?

As was previous mentioned, the goal of a clinical trial is to generate knowledge about whether an intervention can help patients with a disease. As was also previously mentioned, CRM is a methodological science, but it is used to construct experiments that fall into the realm of applied science, and the end results must be such that the results must be useful in clinical practice—that is, the knowledge must be generalizable (have external validity and be actionable). It must have external validity in that the types of patients who are enrolled should not be so specific and homogeneous that the results seen in those patients would be different from those in clinical practice. The characteristics of the patients, intervention, and outcome, must be close enough to clinical practice in order to be transferable to everyday practice.

In addition, the results of the clinical trial must be actionable in that the drug should be given in a fashion that would be practicable in the real world, and the patients must be treated in a similar fashion as they would be in real practice. For example, administration of a drug 6 times a day would not be practicable in clinical practice.

Early Phase Studies

Of course, for Phase I or 2 studies that will be followed by a Phase III study, the performance criteria are somewhat different. For example, practicability and generalizability are less important, since both of these generally will be addressed in Phase III. The study question for early phase studies should be to enable later phase studies, provide clear evidence when a drug candidate is unlikely to ultimately succeed in Phase III, to validate new measurement instruments for Phase III, to provide information to allow appropriate dose selection, and to allow accurate sample size calculation.

2.4 Are Patient Safety and Rights Protected?

The most important constraint—and the most important guiding principle in clinical trial design and conduct—is: do no harm. The key guiding principle should be to protect patient safety. And as was previously mentioned, clinical trials are not conducted for the direct benefit of the enrolled patients. Clinical trials, by definition, are primarily directed toward answering a scientific or clinical question that will benefit the broad group of patients with a disease. The patients in the trial may benefit ultimately, but the trials are in general not designed to maximize the direct benefit to the patients in the trial. Therefore, they must be designed to minimize any potential harm to the patients.

Even the best-designed clinical trials expose patients to risks they would not otherwise have faced, so the scientific and clinical justification for the study must be pristine. There must be scientific equipoise. The lowest (or safest) reasonable dose of the drug, given the goals of the study, must be used. Informed consent must be complete and comprehensible. The monitoring of the study must be close and thorough. Alternate treatment, if withheld, must be withheld only when absolutely necessary and opportunity for rescue medication must be provided.

2.5 Is the Study Parsimonious? Is it Feasible?

In addition, a well-designed study yield not just the right answer but also the maximum quantity and quality of data while utilizing the least amount of resources. CRM is an applied science, and parsimony is an important goal. A well-designed clinical trial enrolls the fewest number of patients necessary to answer the scientific question or hypothesis being tested. In this way, fewest patients are exposed to risk inherent in all clinical trials. Parsimony is achieved by selecting the right group of patients, selecting the appropriate endpoint (that is, for example, sensitive to the treatment effect), and utilizing appropriate statistical analysis.

This is not to say that no data apart from the primary endpoint should be collected. For example, data that identifies any important subgroups that might have a different risk benefit profile compared to the overall tested patient population would be important. This type of data collection should be distinguished from indiscriminate collection of information – this is often wasteful if it is not hypothesis driven, and is often not a good return on the resource used.

The clinical trial should also be feasible. It should be designed so that it can be enrolled, the patients can be compliant, the measurement can be taken, and so on. Sometimes the protocol will have unreasonably narrow inclusion criteria, specify very difficult requirements (such as prohibition of common concomitant medications), or require logistically difficult procedures (such as

FACS analysis within 12 hours of blood collection). In such cases, the trial will often need to be amended or in some cases terminated early. In either case, the validity of the study is affected. Even in cases short of an amendment, the study can become plagued with errors and protocol violations. There are also logistic considerations – for example, it may become prohibitively expensive because of the procedures required.

3 Critical Parameters in Clinical Trial Design

3.1 Design Principles

As was enumerated in the previous section, a well-designed study has to achieve multiple goals: it must have internal and external validity, maximize the likelihood of a positive result, protect patient safety, and be feasible and practicable. In many cases, these priorities are competing, and appropriate trade-offs must be made. For example, making the trial patient population homogeneous might make a positive result more likely and make the study smaller, but it might lessen generalizability and might make enrollment more difficult.

In addition to making appropriate trade-offs, the second major challenge is minimization of biases. This is important in achieving internal validity. For example, the blinding process must be highly rigorous. If there are reactions to the drug administration, side effects, or laboratory parameters that might lead to unblinding, then an appropriate placebo, a blinded assessor, or special blinding procedures are necessary.

Biases can come from outside the study as well. For example, a competing trial enrolling a subset of the patients in question can affect the patient population enrolled. For example, for a myocardial infarction trial taking all comers, if there is a competing trial enrolling only anterior myocardial infarction patients, the resulting enrollment may consist mostly inferior myocardial infarction patients even though the intent was to enroll a representative group of myocardial infarction patients.

Clinical trial hygiene is a critical and difficult aspect of designing and conducting clinical trials. Poor hygiene, such as changing a major inclusion or exclusion criteria in the middle of a study can lead to major, gross bias in the study.

The third challenge is to make sure that the assumptions behind the clinical trial are valid. All clinical trials make assumptions– for example, most trials operate under the assumptions that patients respond independently, that they remain blinded, that dropouts are random, and that clinical practice pattern remains unchanged over time. Making wrong assumptions can lead to failure. For example, if the placebo rate is expected to be 20% on the basis of previous clinical trials, and it turns out to be 30%, then the study may be underpowered to demonstrate a benefit. A common mistake is to assume that the degree of benefit seen in Phase II will be replicated in Phase III. Because of regression to the mean, the effect seen in Phase III will often be less impressive than that seen in Phase II. This is particularly true for escalating dose studies. As another example, if the measurement tool used to assess the endpoint is assumed to have linear response, and if the response turns out to be nonlinear, then the statistical analysis methods may need to be modified.

The fourth, and often the greatest, challenge is to insure that the right question is being asked. No matter how well the trial is designed—even if it does a laudable job of randomization, has appropriate statistical tests, and minimizes other biases—if it asks the wrong question then the study may fail. Each clinical trial is an instance of a particular patient population being treated with a particular dose(s) of the drug, with a particular outcome being measured. If the wrong patients/indication, wrong dose, or wrong endpoint is selected, then the results will be negative, misleading, and/or not generalizable.

3.2 Design Tools

In designing a clinical trial, there are multiple trade-off's and many degrees of freedom. The critical parameters in clinical trial design are the appropriate patient population, the appropriate dose, and the appropriate endpoint. There are other subtleties of clinical trial design that are important, including sample size, blinding, comparator arms, boundary for accepting or rejecting the hypothesis, etc. that are discussed in the following chapters, but these three factors have the greatest impact, and the design choices regarding these are the greatest because there are infinite permutations of patients/doses/endpoints and only a few permutations can be tested.

Implicit in the goal of clinical trials is the assumption that there is a group of subjects who have an undesirable condition (disease) or are at risk of developing an undesirable condition. This brings us to the first step in designing a clinical trial: defining the target and sample populations for the trial. In rare instances, the target population is everyone in the world, such as the target population for the polio vaccine. More typically, it will be necessary to define a group of patients with a set of characteristics and conditions who constitute the target population for the trial. This is the population to whom the results of the study will be generalized or applied. In addition, a group that will be a representative sample drawn from the target population will need to be defined. This is the sample population.

The choice of population, particularly the sample population, is critical. It will determine the likelihood of the intervention showing an effect: if patients whose disease is not responsive to the intervention are included, they could dilute the effect of the intervention. It will determine the ultimate risk-benefit analysis: sicker the group of patients, greater the magnitude of safety issues that can be accepted. The right population will also have an important effect on the practicability of the trial. Narrowing the inclusion criteria, for example, might make internal validity easier to achieve, and might make statistical power greater, but this is often at the expense of generalizability. The appropriate patient population includes patients who are likely to respond to the drug, who will be compliant with therapy, who are homogeneous, and who have an unmet medical need.

Also implicit in clinical trials is the assumption that the difference between the treatment groups can be compared and contrasted. In order to compare the results, at least with the quantitative and statistical tools, it is necessary to measure the outcome. CRM is not a branch of aesthetics. The conclusions are based on manipulation of aggregate data measured and collated in a consistent manner. Therefore, the second critical aspect of clinical trial design is endpoints.

The choice of an appropriate endpoint is perhaps one of the most difficult aspects of clinical trial design. The endpoint must be clinically significant, be responsive to therapy, have low variability, and be representative of the disease status as a whole. Choosing an endpoint that is simple and reductionist might make it easier to determine whether drug exerts an effect on the primary endpoint, but such an endpoint may ignore other clinical parameters and might make generalizability more difficult.

Also implicit in the goal is the assumption that the two comparison groups are two separate groups, uninfluenced by each other. It would make no sense to compare a group to itself. In addition, the assumption is that although the groups are separate, they are groups of similar patients. This is necessary because if there were major underlying differences in the groups, it would be difficult to compare the outcome in the two groups. The groups must be similar enough so that the outcome in the two groups would be similar in absence of intervention. That way, when there is a difference in outcome, the conclusion can be that the intervention caused the difference. Randomization and blinding are two of the ways that this is achieved.

Finally, selection of the appropriate intervention and dose is critical to the success of the trial. Each group of patients should receive a consistent dose or dosing regimen. Comparison between groups would otherwise be impossible. Careful consideration of the dose must be given. Too high of a dose will result in safety issues, and too low of a dose will result in lack of efficacy. Issues such as whether to adjust based on weight, the route of administration, whether to monitor pharmacokinetic/pharmacodynamic, etc. are all critical questions. These issues are addressed in the subsequent sections of this book.

Chapter 3: Measures and Variables

1 Background

1.1 Difference between and Endpoints

No matter what kind of clinical trial — efficacy trial, safety trial, pharmacokinetic trial, pharmacodynamic trial, descriptive trial, or combination of more than one of these—the objective of the trial requires that something be measured, such as blood pressure, walk distance, or levels of drug in plasma. Clinical trials are distinguished from anecdotal case studies in that they draw conclusions based on aggregate data. In order to manipulate and analyze aggregate data, the data must be collected in a quantitative fashion: they must be measured.

The terms "endpoint" and "measure" are terms that are sometimes used loosely in clinical trials. For example, "endpoint" and "measure" are sometimes used to refer to any one of the following:

1. General clinical phenomenon being measured: the general disease or disease characteristic
   - Blood pressure
   - Congestive heart failure

2. Specific clinical phenomenon being measured: an aspect, usually the most significant aspect of a disease
   - Systolic blood pressure
   - Mean blood pressure
   - Exacerbations of congestive heart failure

3. Specific clinical parameter at a specified interval: the aspect of the disease, with a specification regarding duration of observation or follow-up
   - Systolic blood pressure at 12 weeks
   - Congestive heart failure exacerbations over 6 months

4. Specific measure at a specified interval: same as #3, but with specification of the scale used for the measurement
   - Systolic blood pressure at 12 weeks measured in mmHg
   - Number of congestive heart failure exacerbations over 6 months

5. Specific measure at a specified interval, with measurement methods: same as #4, but with detailed method of obtaining the measurement
   - Systolic blood pressure at 12 weeks measured in mmHg, measured after sitting for 5 minutes, repeated 3 times and averaged
   - Number of congestive heart failure exacerbations over 6 months, as defined as need for hospitalization or ER visit

6. Specific measure at a specified interval, with analytic methods: same as #5, but with specification about how the data will be manipulated to draw inferences and conclusions
   - Mean change in systolic blood pressure at 12 weeks compared to baseline measured in mmHg
   - Percentage of patients who had at least 5 mmHg decrease in systolic blood pressure at 12 weeks compared to baseline
   - Frequency of congestive heart failure exacerbations over 6 months, as defined as need for hospitalization or ER visit

7. Specific measure at a specified interval, with analytic methods and comparator group: similar to #6 but specifies a comparator group
   - Mean change in systolic blood pressure at 12 weeks compared to baseline measured in mmHg, compared to placebo
   - Frequency of congestive heart failure exacerbations over 6 months, as defined as need for hospitalization or ER visit, compared to frequency during the previous 6 months

Often, the details of the measure and endpoint are not well described, because sometimes the clinical phenomenon can be measured or characterized in different ways with similar results (for example, many drugs have collinear effects on mean blood pressure and systolic blood pressure so measurement of either yields similar results) or because the researcher chooses to use endpoints that have been used previously by previous researchers. In many cases, this is acceptable.

However, in many other situations, even slight changes in the measurement, the time interval, comparator group, etc. can have a profound effect on the ability of a study to answer the question, the strength of the conclusions that can be drawn, the sample size, and so on. It is therefore imperative that the endpoint and measure be chosen with clear understanding of the implications of the choice.

It is important to distinguish between measure and endpoint. I define "measure" as a numeric, mathematical, or other way of assessing a clinical event or characteristic. Some common measures include mmHg, mortality rate, and number of days in the ICU.

As an analogy, imagine if one were to ask "how far is it from San Francisco to Chicago?" The answer could be expressed in one of a number of ways: in km, in miles, in hours of driving distance, in days of driving distance, in number of zones for the purposes of shipping something by UPS, etc. These are all different ways of measuring how far it is from San Francisco to Chicago. These are different "measures" that can be used to characterize the same phenomena: the distance from San Francisco to Chicago.

Depending on the context, one measure may be better than another. If one were asking the above question because one was shipping a heavy item, the answer in terms of shipping zones would be useful. If one were trying to decide whether one could drive to Chicago in time for a wedding, the answer in terms of driving distance would be the most useful. Similarly, if one wanted to assess the response for a drug that lowered blood pressure, mmHg would be an appropriate measure. If one wanted to know whether high pressure was a risk factor for stroke, simple determination of high blood pressure/normal blood pressure may be sufficient rather than mmHg.

I define "endpoint" as the clinically relevant property that is being measured. For example, "mmHg" is a measure, and "change in mean blood pressure after 6 weeks of therapy" is an endpoint. The measure is used to quantify the endpoint. An endpoint is expressed as a measure that is put in context, with specified time interval and analytical methods.

Extending on the above analogy, the distance between San Francisco and Chicago can be specified as several different things, just as clinical endpoints in a trial can be specified as different things. It can be from downtown to downtown, geographic center to geographic center, from airport to airport, etc. It can also be specified as: driving time if one kept to the speed limit, driving time if one were transporting a manufactured home and had to drive at 55 mph, driving time with a radar detector, etc. In a clinical trial, an endpoint can be difference in blood pressure after 6 weeks, the highest recorded blood pressure at any point during 6 weeks, absolute blood pressure after 12 weeks of therapy, etc. As will be discussed in the next chapter, specifying the endpoint is an extremely important aspect of clinical trial design.

Measure can be thought of as the bricks and endpoints as houses or buildings. However, measures can also be used for other purposes – for example, to stratify patients, and to adjust results of analysis in a multivariate model—just as bricks can be used for other purposes, such as building roads.

Measure is a component of an endpoint, and so it is critical to understand measures before discussing endpoints.

1.2 Challenges in Measures

Precise, reproducible, and accurate measurements are not always easy. There are many factors that can pose obstacles to measurements, including but not limited to the following.

- Variability in the presentation of a disease – such as lupus – or protean manifestations of the disease
- Waxing and waning disease – psoriasis, for example can wax and wane on its own
- Training effect – for example, patients who perform treadmill tend to get conditioned over time and perform better on later tests than on the first
- Placebo effect
- Inter-observer variability – for example, different observers may assign different TIMI scores to the same flow on an angiogram
- Different definitions of the disease – for example, what may be considered asthma by one physician may be classified as COPD by another
- Effects of geography and seasons – for example, sunlight may improve psoriasis, or allergens during allergic season might exacerbate rhinitis
- Carry-over effect in subjective diagnosis – for example, for subjective measurements such as PASI, the score may be affected by the severity of the disease in a recent unrelated patient who was seen recently seen by the physician
- Unmasking of the drug and placebo from pain or other side effects of the drug
- Unmasking from the efficacy of the drug
- Defects in instrument or measurement methods

Some of these factors can be ameliorated by blinding and randomization, and others by logistic solutions such as core labs and site training. For others, the best way of ameliorating these issues is through good clinical trial design, and selection of a good measure.

The key properties (or performance characteristics) of a good measure are

- It accurately reflects the phenomenon being measured (is accurate)
- It has low variability and is repeatable (is precise)
- It is sensitive/responsive (is rich in information and yields a good distribution of values in a population of patients)

In addition, for the purposes of clinical trials, a good measure also should have the following properties

- It measures something that is relevant – usually clinical relevant
- It should not influence response or otherwise have biological effect in and of itself

A measure that satisfies these requirements will be reliable, practicable, and allow reliable and informative conclusions to be drawn. These and other aspects of measures are discussed in this chapter.

2 Accuracy and Precision

2.1 Definitions

Two of the key requirements for a good measure are accuracy and precision.

Accuracy refers to how well the measure reflects the phenomenon being measured. In other words, are there any systematic biases? For example, how well does calculated glomerular filtration rate (glomerular filtration rate) correspond to true glomerular filtration rate?

A measurement that is precise but not accurate yields values that are very close to each other on measurement after measurement but the numbers are consistently off. An example would be measuring blood pressure with a state of the art instrument, but with a small cuff on a patient with a large arm. The blood pressure readings will consistently be higher than the true value. No matter how many times the measurement is repeated, it will not be possible to correct this error, because the error is not random – it's systematic.

Precision refers to how reproducible the measurement is – if we measured glomerular filtration rate ten times on a patient as a given time, would the values be very similar to each other? Or will there be a lot of random variation – large variability?

A measurement that is not precise but accurate is an endpoint with a lot of variability. An example would be blood pressure measured with an instrument that had a very small display, and was marked only with 10 mmHg increments so that it was difficult to distinguish between measurements that were less than 10 mmHg apart – one would have to estimate the mmHg. A measurement that lacks precision is said to have a lot of *variability*. An imprecise measure can be overcome by repeating the measurement multiple times and taking the average. Each measurement may be slightly wrong but the direction of the error is random so by averaging a large number of measurements, it's possible to determine at the true value.

These concepts are illustrated below.

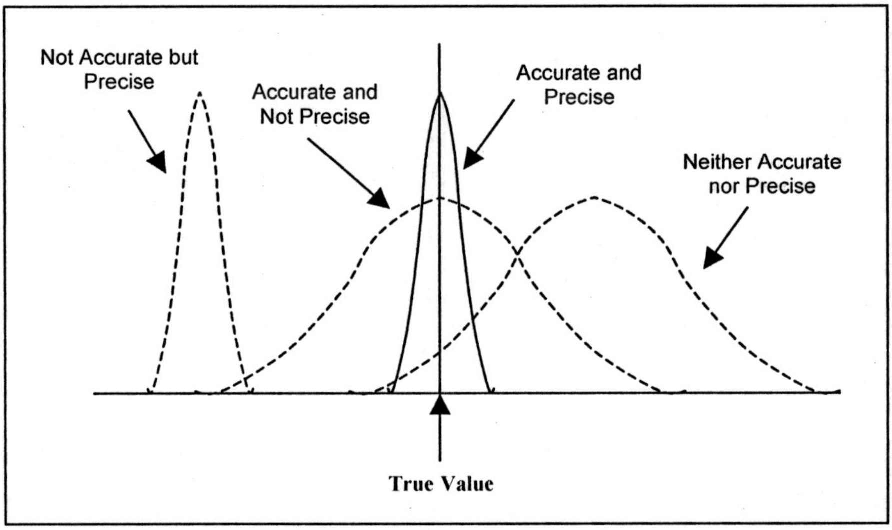

2.2 Consequences of Poor Accuracy and Precision

One of the most important consequences of poor precision (also called lack or reliability, lack of repeatability, or high variability) is an increase in sample size required to answer the scientific question. Given that a cardinal responsibility of a clinical researcher is to answer the research question in the most parsimonious (not in the economic sense but in the scientific sense) fashion possible, maximizing precision is critical.

It is often thought that poor precision can always be compensated for by an increase in sample size. To a large degree this is true, particularly when the measure is being used as an endpoint. However, apart from the fact that it is not always feasible to increase the sample size, there are consequences of poor precision that cannot be ameliorated simply with increase in sample size.

As an example, if there is poor precision in the measure that is used to determine eligibility into the study, then patients not likely to benefit or perhaps even suffer detriment from the therapy may be enrolled. An example would be enrollment of patients without diabetes into a study of anti-hyperglycemic agents, because the measure used to determine whether the patients had diabetes had poor precision. If the endpoint were all-cause hospitalization or death, the inclusion of such patients might make the results negative. In that case, even an increase in sample size may not be enough to salvage the study. Certainly, at a minimum, the estimate of the effect size will be erroneous. In this particular case, poor precision in the measure used for inclusion criteria has an impact on the accuracy (external validity) of the study as a whole. Exactly the same issue exists when a measure with poor precision is used to segregate the study population for subgroup analysis.

Poor accuracy has even more dire consequences. An endpoint with poor accuracy will lead to a biased result, and may make the results of the study meaningless.

2.3 Precision and Variability

2.3.1 Sources of Precision Error/Variability

As was previously mentioned, precision is lost when there is an increase in random error. There are three main sources for random error, at least when the measurement is in a static item (not separated by time), as enumerated by Hulley and summarized below.[1] Each of these can be separated further into intra (within the same patient, observer, or instrument) and inter (between patients, observer, or instruments) types. The distinction between intra and inter variability is important insofar as the tactics used to reduce the two type of variability differ. For example, by specifying that same physician conduct the joint exam on every patient will reduce inter-observer variability on the ACR 20 score but not intra-observer variability.

Subject variability is the first source. Some examples include the following.

Intra-patient variability examples:
- Motivation of the patient (treadmill, visual acuity chart, FEV1)
- Patient mistakes (misunderstanding directions, marking wrong box on questionnaire)

Inter-patient variability examples:

- Heterogeneity due to gender, ethnic background, etc.
- Different concomitant conditions (degree of PAD or osteoarthritis on ability to complete ETT)

Observer variability is the second source. Some examples include

Intra-observer variability examples:
- Time spent on exam (likelihood of detecting new murmur)
- Estimating the area of body surface area covered by plaques

Inter-observer variability examples:
- Different local standards in hospitalizing patient
- Difference in estimating TIMI flow
- Differences in how the patients are instructed (when the patient is allowed to stop the ETT)

Instrument variability is the third source. Some examples include the following.

Intra-instrument variability examples:
- Variability of the viral assay from batch to batch
- Effect of humidity or vibration in instrument
- Variability in the speed of the treadmill from one ETT to next

Inter-instrument variability examples:
- Differences in calibration between different manufacturers (ECHO machine, MRI's)

These errors decrease the precision of measurement, and every effort to minimize these errors should be taken. Some of the strategies are discussed below.

In addition, it is important to characterize and document the precision of measurements used in clinical trials. Imprecise measures can significantly weaken the ability to draw conclusions from a study.

It's important to note that although variability due to imprecise measures is an important source of variability in clinical trial and has a major impact on the sample size, there are other factors that affect variability, and there are other factors besides variability that impact sample size. The table below summarizes some of the most common ones.

Other Sources of Variability

The discussion in this section is not part of measurement; however, it is closely linked to precision.

Although the factors discussed in the previous section capture most of the sources of variability in a static measure, additional factors contribute to variability when measures are repeated over time. These are summarized below.

Disease status change:
An important source of variability is change in the disease or clinical condition over time. Diseases such as multiple sclerosis and psoriasis wax and wane over time. Levels of cortisol levels vary over the course of a day.

Environmental change:
As seasons change, changes in pollen levels can have an effect on the disease. For example, when a patient move from Maine to Florida, his UV exposure increases, which can improve psoriasis.

Differences in intervention:
Different batches of the drug, particularly biologics, can have different potency. Differences in compliance can also increase variability.

Differences in response:
Depending on the (sub) types of disease (classic AMD *vs.* occult AMD) or patient characteristics (HER2 positive *vs.* negative), different patients can have differential response to the drug.

Variability in background therapy or concomitant treatment/medications:
In different parts of the world for example, the patients may be subject to different therapies.

All of these factors increase variability and therefore sample size. These should be distinguished from factors that can introduce bias, such as unblinding or poor blinding, which can introduce a differential effect between the active and placebo groups. These are to be avoided as well, but are different from increases in variability.

2.3.2 Measuring Precision

The simplest measurement of precision is simply the standard deviation (SD) in a sample. Larger the SD, less precise the measurement is. SD can be divided by the mean to yield coefficient of variation, which is a unit-less measure than can be used to compare precision. For example, if something is measure in cm and another in inches, coefficient of variation can be used to compare precision.

A better way of characterizing precision is to compare consistency across two or more sets of measurements, such as test-retest consistency and inter-observer consistency.

The below figure illustrates two sets of tests – such as two sets of blood pressure measurements on the same population. A highly precise test would be expected to have most of the measurements on the diagonal line. There are several ways to statistically express the precision, but the most common ones are:

- Correlation coefficient: the closeness of the fit to the diagonal line plus the rank order of the measurements
- Standard (typical) error of measurement: standard deviation of the error of the measurement, or the closeness of the fit to the diagonal line, rank order is not considered, and less prone to sampling bias
- Change in mean: change in the mean between the first and second measurement
- Kappa coefficient: similar to correlation coefficient, but for nominal variables

Measuring Precision: two sets of measurements graphed against each other

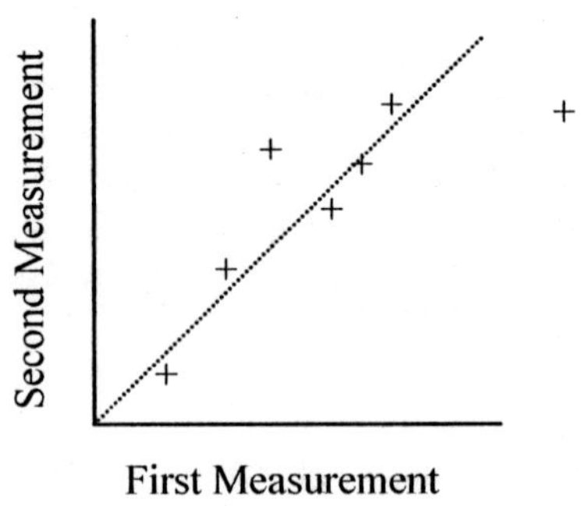

Below are some specific types of precision measurements. The degree of precision required of a measurement is dependent on external factors such as

the goals of the clinical trial, maximal feasible sample size, and other similar considerations.

Test-Retest Consistency:

A measurement can be repeated multiple times on the same set of patients. This can be used to establish replicability of a measurement. Care should be exercised regarding the timing between retesting. For some, such as blood pressure, the test can be done immediately. Others such as visual acuity chart may have a carryover effect so it is advisable to wait before retesting in such cases. On the other hand, waiting too long could allow a change in the parameter being measured – for example, visual acuity might truly change after a month.

Intraobserver Consistency:

The same observer might perform the retest, in which case intraobserver consistency would be measured. To control for patient variability, it is preferable to have the observer measure the same patients or samples on retests. An ideal example would be to use the same set of photographs or ECG's.

Inter-observer Consistency:

Similarly, multiple observers can be asked to evaluate the same set of patients or the same photograph/ECG, etc. and the correlation between their observations can be described.

Internal Consistency:

Internal consistency can be established by using similar ways of measuring a phenomenon. For example, blood pressure obtained noninvasively with a spygnomanometer and blood pressure obtained invasively with an arterial line, can be compared, and they should correlate with each other.

2.4 Accuracy and Validity

2.4.1 Sources of Accuracy Error/Bias

When error occurs with regard to accuracy, it is called bias. Decrease in accuracy is caused by systematic, not random, error, such that the measurement is consistently off in one direction. Sources for accuracy error can be classified into three categories, as with precision errors, but there are no distinctions between intra and inter types of errors (since all errors are between the measure and true value). These have also been enumerated by Hulley and summarized below.[1]

Subject bias is the first source. Some examples include

- Placebo effect
- Recall bias (patient tends to recall being exposed to asbestos better than being exposed to something innocuous like orchids)
- "White Coat Effect" (BP higher when measured in the office)

Observer bias is the second source. Some examples include

- Physician might overestimate response if he believes in the efficacy of the drug
- Physician might underreport adverse events if he tend to be rushed in his assessments

Instrument bias is the third source. Some example include

- Screening test with low sensitivity will underestimate incidence of a disease
- Uncalibrated instrument may drift over time, yielding high or low value

Other Sources of Bias

There are multiple other sources of bias, including unblinding, the fact that a patients enrolled in a clinical trial receive closer medical care, and training/conditioning.

As with variability, every effort should be taken to minimize bias.

It's important to note that although bias due to inaccurate measure is an important source of bias in the trial and has a major impact on the conclusions of the study and the generalizability to the broader population, there are other factors that affect bias.

2.4.2 Assessing Accuracy and Validity

2.4.2.1 Overview

Accuracy can be considered to be a measure of validity (although strictly speaking, validity requires good accuracy plus either good precision or large sample size). Validity is the ability to measure the phenomena that one is intending to measure. Validity doesn't exist in isolation but only in context of the intended phenomena being measured, the intended population, and for the intended purpose.

Measures used in clinical trials must be validated. Unvalidated measures make clinical trial results meaningless because there is no assurance that the results reflect clinical phenomenon. Unvalidated measures are unacceptable in clinical research.

Validity is a term that is rife with confusion, and is used in many different ways by different people, and the types of validity also are a matter of debate. However, one can categorize three possible methods of assessing or establishing accuracy as discussed below. Most of the discussion below is based on work by Trochim.[2]

2.4.2.2 Validate against a Gold Standard (Criterion Validity)

The first is to validate the measure against one or more other accepted measures. If the comparison is against a "Gold Standard," this is called establishing criterion validity. For example, if biopsy proven rejection is the accepted standard for transplant rejection, and we wish to establish that a blood marker X is a good measure of rejection, data demonstrating that it correlates well (high specificity and sensitivity) with biopsy results could can establish its accuracy. In this way, the blood marker could become a validated way of measuring the same phenomena – namely, rejection.

The measures of validity are similar to the measures of precision: validation correlation, errors of the estimate, and kappa coefficient.

2.4.2.3 Validate against Other Outcome Measures (Criterion-Related Validity)

If a gold standard doesn't exist, the second way of establishing accuracy or validity is through the following. Ideally, all of the following should be satisfied.

Predictive Validity:

Predictive validity is demonstration that the measure is predictive of or correlated with an outcome (sometimes called predictive or construct validity). For example, even if the blood marker X has poor or moderate correlation with biopsy proven rejection, if it correlates better with graft loss in 12 months than the biopsy, it could be established as a valid measure that predicts an outcome. It would not be validated necessarily as a way of measuring rejection *per se* if it doesn't correlate with biopsy proven rejection, but could be a valid measure of a phenomena that was clinically relevant.

In many instances, it is easier to define a dichotomous outcome, such as rejection or death, and from it derive a prior continuous outcome as something that correlates with the likelihood of the dichotomous outcome, because the dichotomous outcome is sometime more definitive or easier to determine – for example, death. In some instances, however, a dichotomous outcome is soft – such as a lupus flare. In that case, it may be necessary to rely on the method below.

Concurrent Validity:

Concurrent validity is the ability of the measure to correlate with another measure of the phenomena. Criterion validity is a form of concurrent validity.

Postdictive Validity:

Postdictive validity is the ability of the measure to distinguish between what it's measuring and other phenomena that happened in the past. For example, the blood marker X should correlate with other prior predictors of rejection such as unrelated donor transplant, prior noncompliance, etc.

Construct Validity:

Construct validity a loose term, but means that the overall set of correlations among measures seem to make sense. In a way, construct validity is akin to multivariate modeling, compared to predictive, concurrent, or postdictive validity which are more like univariate modeling. I define construct validity as the sum of convergent validity and divergent validity.

When the comparison is to a set of measures that are expected to correlate with the measure, this is convergent validity. For example, even if biopsy results are not available, if the blood marker X results correlate with need for increased immunosuppression, decreased glomerular filtration rate, etc., then it may be possible to establish validity. Convergent validity is similar to concurrent validity but convergent validity requires correlation with multiple other measures, and the other measures do not measure the same phenomena. Rather, they measure other phenomena that in theory should be related to the phenomena of interest (for example, measures compliance with meds, not rejection directly).

Divergent validity (sometimes called discriminate validity) is opposite of convergent validity. For instance, blood marker X should be negatively correlated with successful transplantation, need to increased immunosuppression, etc., and poorly correlated with incidence of osteoarthritis, myopia, etc.

2.4.2.4 Assert Accuracy of the Measure as an Axiom (Face and Content Validity)

The third way of establishing accuracy or validity is to take an endpoint that has clear clinical relevance, such as visual acuity, and to assert that it is accurate (sometimes called face or content validity). Alternatively, a consensus conference can establish a measure (such as ACR or congestive heart failure classification) as an acceptable endpoint (consensual validity).

Face validity is whether the measure appears to be reasonable. It is a very general criterion – for example, joint count appears to be a reasonable measure of joint involvement in RA. Content validity is whether a certain criteria is met by the measure – for example, does the ACR20 score meet the prespecified criteria set by ACR: correlation with expert opinions, correlation with response to methotrexate, etc.?

If a measure is being asserted as being a valid measure *de novo*, it is optimal to demonstrate that the measure has acceptable precision. It would be helpful also to show that the measure is sensitive and practical.

2.5 Improving Precision and Accuracy (Minimizing Variability and Bias)

Variability and bias can be reduced by the following methods.

Training sites:

Example: holding an investigator's meeting to train study site personnel and making site visits to insure that the study coordinators and physicians at the sites are well trained in the use of equipment and the instructions for measurement

Detailed instructions:

Example: issuing specific instructions on how to perform the measurements outlined in the protocol, such as angle to hold the ultrasound, number of photographs to be taken, how long to leave the tourniquet on, etc.

Trial runs:

Example: having study sites send in test samples/ECG's/ECHO's to insure that they can perform high quality measurements.

Core laboratory:

Example: processing laboratory samples, and having readings of ECG, MRI, etc. performed at a core laboratory with appropriate procedures. At a minimum, the readings should be repeated by two or more readers. There should also be written discrepancy resolution procedures, full documentation, full audit trail, etc.

Multiple measurements:

For measurements that are relatively easy to perform, such as blood pressure, performing several measurements and averaging the results or discarding out the highest and lowest values

Run-in phase:
For measures prone to conditioning or training, such as treadmill or visual acuity charts, a run-in period to train the patient before true measurements are obtained. Also, run-in phase can be helpful to eliminate placebo responders, or to eliminate nonresponders.

Insuring instrument calibration:

Example: specifying the window during which the instrument had to have been calibrated or sending samples to sites to run on their machine

Using same equipment:

Example: providing or specifying the type of equipment, assay reagent, etc.

Using better equipment:

Using higher quality or later generation equipment, such as third generation optical coherence imaging

Automating equipment:

Example: using the built-in algorithms for cardiac output on MUGA scans, etc.

Adjudication of events:

For some clinical events that are so complex as to require clinical evaluation, an adjudication committee may be required to evaluate clinical events – such as intracranial hemorrhage

Unobtrusive measurements:

Making unobtrusive measurements minimize the likelihood that the measurement itself will affect outcome.

Improving the blinding of the placebo:

Using same color inert ingredient, same pH (so that it stings the same amount as active ingredient), covering the IV bag to mask color, etc.

Sham procedures:

Example: sham intravitreal injections in age-related macular degeneration studies, where placebo injection would be unethical due to risk of endophthalmitis

Blinded assessor:

Where unblinding is possible, using blinded assessor to perform efficacy measurements such as ACR. The blinded assessor is usually a separate physician than the treating physician, and not permitted to communicate with each other regarding the study. Alternatively, using a blinded safety assessor in cases where certain unblinding information is critical to insure patient safety. An example would be an immunosuppressive drug study in transplant patients where an unblinded safety assessor might follow hematological parameters.

Blind unblinding variables:

Having an unblinded investigator view all potential unblinding data, and having a separate blinded investigator perform the assessments. Examples include PTT for heparin and lymphocyte count for cellular trafficking inhibitors.

Compliance Tools:

Example: increase levels of compliance and monitor compliance with pill counts or with electronic pill counters that can be built into the study drug container.

3 Types of Measures/Variables

3.1 Overview

When something is measured, it yields a value, such as 177 cm, 14 kg, black, white, true, or false. These values can be numbers or non-numbers. There are several different types of values that a measure can yield: a measure can be one of several different types of variables. These categories (sometimes called scales of variables) are described below.

These categories are extremely important in clinical trials because the type of variable that is used as an endpoint has a profound impact on power/sample size of the trials and the clinical relevance of the results. For example, the exact quantitative glomerular filtration rate is more informative than a yes/no value regarding the presence or absence of renal failure. Also, they have an important impact on the robustness of the study to dropouts (patients who discontinue the study) and missing values.

Also, richer variables are more informative and useful when used as a covariate or when used to divide and analyze patients in subgroups. For example, a quantitative variable, such as age, is much more informative than a qualitative variable such as adult (over 18 yrs old)/non-adult. If someone is an adult, they might be 18, 40, or 80 years old – in and of itself "adult" doesn't convey nearly as much information as "33 years old."

To expand on this, a statement, "Adults in the study had 3% incidence of bleeding in this study and children had 1% incidence" is not nearly as informative as "Subjects who were 0-10 years old had 0% bleeding, 10-20 had 2%, 20-40 had 4.5% and 40-80 had 10%," or "For each additional year, the risk of bleeding increased by 0.2%."

The more values a variable can have, higher the information content. The types of variables are summarized in the table below, and discussed in detail in the sections that follow.

Types of Measures/Variables		
Type		
Qualitative	Nominal	
	Ordinal	
Quantitative	Interval Discrete	Interval Continuous
	Ratio Discrete	Ratio Continuous

3.2 Quantitative Variables

The most important distinction between different types of variables is between quantitative (numeric) and categorical (or non-quantitative, sometime called qualitative) variables.

Quantitative variables are variables such as weight, height, or age, that can be added, subtracted, and otherwise mathematically manipulated. Categorical variables are variables such as hair color, death/survival, geography, etc. that are different from one another but cannot be added, subtracted, or mathematically manipulated. Categorical variables are sometimes called qualitative variables, but this term can be confusing in clinical trials because "qualitative" has a different meaning in colloquial medical usage: usually it means subjective rather than objective measures. Because of this potential confusion, I will use "categorical" to refer to non-quantitative variables.

Because quantitative variables, especially continuous variables (see below) contain so much more information than categorical variables, samples sizes of studies can be influenced tremendously by choice of the variable type. For example, a wound healing trial using "healed/non-healed" categorical variable (in other words, the response is categorized simply as healed or not healed) might require hundreds of patients, whereas one using continuous variable of "percentage area healed" might require tens of patients to achieve the same degree of statistical power.

Similarly, average change in blood pressure or average change in PASI score tends to be more informative than whether blood pressure normalized or whether a patient had a complete remission of his psoriasis symptoms.

Example:

In a diabetic wound healing trial, the quantitative variable of area of healing is much more informative than the qualitative (non-quantitative) variable of healed/not healed. For example, if the results were that placebo arm had 3/10 patients heal their wounds *vs.* 5/10 in the treated arm, it would be difficult to draw strong conclusions. If, however, the same results are presented as 25% average healing n the placebo arm *vs.* 90% in the treated arm, this would be much more informative. It would be similarly informative if there were 45% average healing in the placebo arm and 55% in the treated arm. The key point is that 3/10 *vs.* 5/10 could be either of these two possibilities: qualitative variables generally don't convey as much information as quantitative variables.

Because quantitative variables contain more information than categorical variables, they can be converted to categorical variables, but the reverse is not true. For example, blood pressure can be categorized in low, normal or high. Tumor response can be classified as no response, partial response, or complete response, etc. But "low" blood pressure cannot be converted into a specific mmHg measure without additional information.

Quantitative variables can be continuous or discrete.

3.2.1 Continuous Variables

Continuous variables are variables such as age or blood pressure that can be subdivided into infinitely smaller gradations – such as 3.5 years, 3.75 years, etc. They are real numbers (as opposed to integers).

3.2.2 Discrete Variables

Discrete (also called count) variables are usually integer variables like number of exacerbations or number of prior pregnancies. These variables cannot be subdivided. A convenient way to tell continuous variables from discrete variables is that continuous variables always have some unit of measurement such as year, degrees Celsius, etc. while discrete variable do not (though they may have names – such as "number of pregnancies") have units of measurement.

Continuous variables contain more information than discrete variables so they can be converted into discrete variables but not the other way around (This is an important factor to remember when designing case report forms – you can derive lower information variables from high information variables but not vice-versa.).

To reiterate, the distinguishing feature of quantitative variables is that they can be added, subtracted, averaged, and otherwise mathematically manipulated and still retain meaning. This is not true for categorical variables such as eye color – it is not meaningful to add black and brown eyes and divide by blue eyes for example.

In clinical trials, it is extremely important to recognize that not every numeric measure is a true quantitative variable. For example, one cannot add or divide renal tubular acidosis type I, II, III, and IV or congestive heart failure class I, II, III, and IV. They are represented numerically but are in fact categorical variables. Similarly, although ACR20, ACR50, etc. appear on face to be quantitative variables, they cannot (or should not) be manipulated numerically.

3.2.3 Approximating Quantitative Variables in Clinical Practice

On the other hand, most biological phenomena are not strictly linear and yet we treat many variables as continuous variables when in fact they are, strictly speaking, approximations of continuous variables. We commonly do this particularly with composite scores such as PASI scores – with PASI, we treat 1% of the body surface area covered with erythema as being equivalent to 1% of the surface area being covered by a plaque. This is clearly an approximation. It is partially because many variables used in clinical practice are actually approximations of a quantitative variable that some clinicians and the FDA prefer dichotomous variables to continuous variables.

It should be noted that even for variables that are continuous such as blood pressure, the biological significance over a broad range of values may not be linear. For example, a 10 mmHg difference may have different clinical significance depending on whether it represents the difference between 75 and 85, 115 and 125, or 260 and 270 mmHg. Similarly, 6 month increase in survival has different significance for a patient with life expectancy of 2 months versus someone with a life expectancy of 50 years, so it's probably not appropriate to utilize averages for all clinical situations even if the variable is truly quantitative. (In some cases, if the clinical significance is exponential or other mathematically regular function, it may be possible to transform it mathematically to yield a continuous variable).

A subset of quantitative variables is also "ratio" variables – that is, absolute 0 means something and doubling the value doubles the meaning of the value. Age is a true ratio variable. Temperature expressed in degrees Celsius is an example of a variable that is not a ratio variable – doubling the temperature doesn't mean that something is twice as hot. Degrees expressed in degrees Kelvin, on the other hand, is a ratio variable. Ratio variables and interval variables (non-ratio) can be used in clinical trials without significant impact on trial design.

3.3 Categorical Variables

In many clinical trials, categorical variables are employed to construct endpoints. Often, this is because they are the most clinical relevant endpoints – for example, death/survival is a very important categorical variable. In other instances, the regulatory agencies will insist on categorical variables because they want to set a high bar and/or want the clinical significance to be clear.

An average relative change of 50% in PASI score, for example, or average absolute change of 10% in ejection fraction, for example, can be difficult to interpret. 50% change in PASI might occur in a patient going from a score of 10 to a 5 or from 60 to 30. Difference of 10% in ejection fraction is different in someone who starts with an ejection fraction of 20% versus someone who starts with an ejection fraction of 50%.

Mean change is also difficult to interpret because even with a mean improvement of 10% in ejection fraction, some patients might have had 25% change and other -5% change.

Clinical significance is most clear if absolute cut-off for baseline and post-treatment is set. Example would be proportion of patients who start with ejection fraction below 20% and end with an ejection fraction of greater than 40% or proportion of patients who start with FEV_1 below 60% and end with FEV_1 greater than 80%. These are high bars with clear clinical meaning.

Next in clinical significance is the proportion of patients with large absolute or relative change in disease, such as substantial change in PASI or exercise tolerance test (ETT) time. (This is to be distinguished from large change in average PASI or ETT). For example, percentage of patients who increase their visual acuity by 3 lines or more would be of clear clinical significance.

Next in clinical significance are patients who start above a threshold and end up below a threshold. An example would be the percentage of patients who were unable to walk unassisted before the treatment but are able to walk after.

3.3.1 Ordinal Variables

Categorical variables can be ordinal or nominal. Ordinal (or rank) variables are variables that have an order of significance, such complete response, partial response, and non-response. In such a case, one variable is clearly better or greater than another. Another example would be categories of congestive heart failure: Class I, II, III, and IV. One category is better than another, but it's not meaningful to add or average the values.

3.3.2 Nominal Variables

Nominal variables are variables that do not have a meaningful order, such as northern region, southern region, and northwestern region, or ragweed/peanut/cat allergies. Each value of a nominal variable must be mutually exclusive of others and the set of variables must be exhaustive. In other words, there must not be any gaps in the categories –for example, Hawaii must be included in the geographic classification, one cannot define adults as >21 and children as <18 without having a category for 18-21. Nor should one define adults as >18 and children as <21.

3.3.3 Dichotomous Variables

Dichotomous variables are variable that have only two possible values, such as dead/alive, true/false, responder/nonresponder.

---

[1] Hulley, SB, Cummings SR. *Designing Clinical Research.* Baltimore, Williams & Wilkins, 1988.

[2] Trochim WMK. *The Research Methods Knowledge Base.* Cincinnati, Atomicdog publishing, 2001.

Chapter 4: Endpoints

1 Background

As was discussed in the previous chapter, the terms "endpoint" and "measure" are terms that are sometimes used loosely in clinical trials. As a reminder, I defined "measure" as the method of assessing a clinical phenomena, and endpoint as the clinical phenomena being measured.

Earlier, it was discussed how the answer to the question "how far is it from San Francisco to Chicago" depends on the specific definition being used, such as downtown to downtown, airport to airport, driving at 55 mph, etc. Similarly, in clinical trials, it is critical to specify the exact clinical phenomena being measured.

Each of the major parameters in the construct of an endpoint is discussed in detail below, but there are several key characteristics of a good clinical endpoint.

First, it must accurately and comprehensively reflect the overall disease being treated. Or in other words, it should be relevant to the clinical question being asked. For example, if the disease being treated were systemic lupus erythematosus (SLE), then an endpoint that only focuses on skin manifestations would not be a good endpoint because other manifestations of lupus may be missed. If the intent of the therapy were to improve overall status of a patient with SLE, this would be an inappropriate endpoint. On the other hand, if the drug is only intended to improve skin manifestations, the endpoint may be acceptable.

Second, it should capture sufficient and appropriate information to allow aggregate analysis that will allow the investigator or sponsor to draw appropriate conclusions. Except for few situations, it is preferable to capture endpoints with richer information than less. For example, if a drug is meant to induce remission in mild Crohn's disease, then the endpoint should be within 8-12 weeks, not after 6 months since the rate of natural remission would be similar to that of an effective therapy at 6 months. If the drug is meant to reduce the size of infarct after a myocardial infarction, then the endpoint should characterize the ejection fraction in terms of percent ejection fraction not in terms of normal *vs.* reduced ejection fraction.

The choice of endpoint also has a profound effect on the likelihood of a positive clinical trial result. An appropriate endpoint, that is sensitive to treatment effect and contains enough information to discriminate between a group that is responding and the group that isn't, is critical to the success of a clinical trial. (Of course, in addition, there must be enough patients in the trial, the drug must have enough of a biological effect, and the measurement must be sensitive enough for the study to be adequately powered.)

Characteristics of a Good Endpoint

- It measures something that is relevant – usually clinically relevant
- It is responsive and rich in information – sensitive, discriminating, and has good distribution
- It is reliable (is precise, has low variability, and reproducible) even across studies
- It should be as robust to dropouts and missing data as possible
- It should not influence response or otherwise have biological effect in and of itself
- Is practical (can be implemented at different sites, and must be measurable in all patients, and is economical, and is noninvasive, preferably)

Third, the endpoint should be reproducible and verifiable. For example, if an echocardiogram is used, then specific instructions on the settings, mode, etc. should be specified so that an independent technician could reproduce the procedure in the same way. The echocardiograms should be recorded and archived (or better yet, sent to a Core Lab) so that the reading could be double checked, and compared against other echocardiograms if necessary.

Fourth, the endpoint should be robust to dropouts and missing data. For example, all-cause mortality is relatively robust to a few dropouts because the imputation can be done as worst case and the dropouts counted as deaths. However, frequency of flare is not robust to dropout because it is extremely difficult to impute the flare rates for the patients who drop out during the study.

There are a few other considerations, such as the requirement that the act of collecting the endpoint should not in and of itself have a biological effect or affect the endpoint itself, but these are discussed in more detail below.

2 Clinical Relevance

2.1 Overview

One of the most important aspects of selecting and defining an endpoint is its clinical relevance. The most sensitive and reliable measure is of little use if the results do not have clinical meaning, or can be extrapolated to an endpoint that has clinical meaning.

Clinical relevance is dependent on several factors, including importance of the endpoint being measured, the magnitude of the change, and functional outcome. Ultimately, the clinical relevance of the endpoint is linked to things that matter to the patient.

Classically, symptoms are considered to be the most important to the patients, and by extension, the most clinically relevant endpoints. This is in contrast to signs or surrogate laboratory measures, which are generally considered to be less clinically relevant. These are usually reasonable assumptions.

However, the true value of an endpoint is not symptoms themselves but the emotive component of it. Symptoms generally elicit feelings in patients, and when the feelings have a negative emotive component, such that patients do not want to experience the symptoms, that represent the true essence of clinical relevance.

Because patients often have emotive feelings attached to common diagnosis, the signs and diagnosis associated with a disease can sometimes become a highly clinically relevant endpoint, such as with myocardial infarction (heart attack to the patient).

It is important to distinguish between symptoms from the emotive response to the symptoms, because different patients have different emotive reactions to similar symptoms. Also, in some cases, an intervention may affect the emotive response to the symptom without affecting the symptoms itself. For example, with pain, symptom of pain may be dissociated from the emotive effects. In rare conditions, a patient may still feel the pain but without any negative emotive association with it. A drug, such as ziconotide, that decrease the negative emotive component may be considered to have a true clinical effect even if the effect on a traditional pain scale such as Visual Analog Scale of Pain Intensity (VASPI) is moderate.

These types of effects should be distinguished from drugs that are directed solely toward the symptom itself. An example might be a drug such as diazepam that might reduce the symptoms of atrial fibrillation without affecting the atrial fibrillation itself.

Pyramid of Clinical Relevance

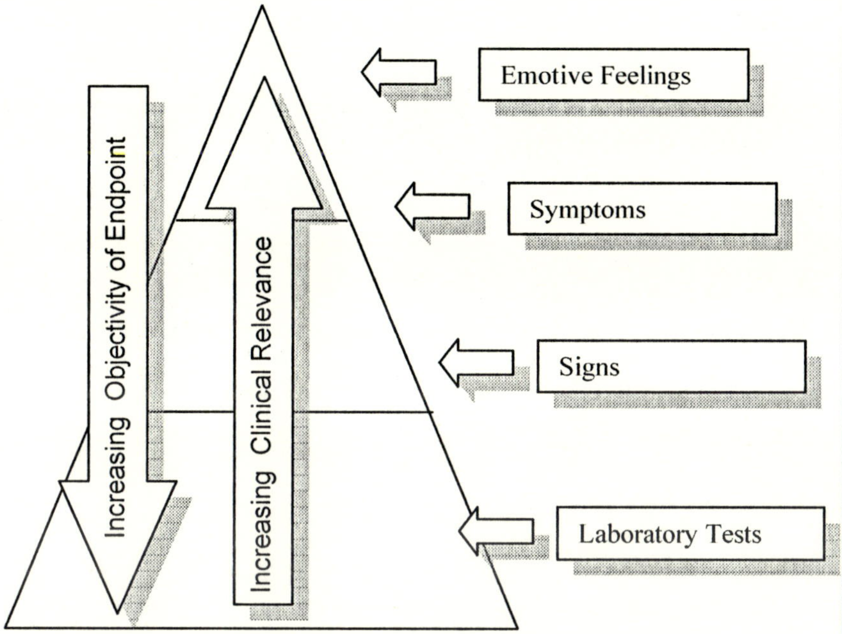

Emotive Feelings: How patients feel about their symptoms and disease. Captured as Quality of Life or Patient Reported Outcome measures

Symptoms: What patients feel, such as pain, dizziness, shortness of breath. Sometimes captured as Quality of Life, sometimes as clinical endpoint.

Signs: Observations by physician or other personnel, such as cough, skin rash, or heart murmur. This is the most common level of clinical endpoint measurements.

Laboratory Test: Surrogate measurements such as radiograph, ECG, or blood count. Generally this is the most objective measurement, but least clinically relevant.

Unfortunately, however, symptoms are difficult to measure and quantify, and emotive response to the symptoms are even more difficult. Signs and laboratory measurements tend to be more objective and easier to quantify, but at the cost of clinical relevance. Clinical endpoints rely on a mixture of measurements, but the dominant components of endpoints in clinical studies are usually signs and diagnosis. Signs and diagnosis occur at the level of the physician, and includes things such as joint count, multiple sclerosis relapse, and renal failure. It can also include other objective measures that are the consequence of a physician's clinical judgement such as hospitalizations.

In addition, clinical relevance is determined by the magnitude of effect as well. Some studies may show a statistical difference between the control and the active groups, but the difference may be too small to be of clinical relevance. For example, a drug might reduce length of hospitalization by 2 hours on average, and this could be statistically significant if the study was large enough.

It might seem that the simplest, most clinically relevant endpoint is a cure or a remission. That way, there is no question about whether the endpoint is linear or continuous, and the clinical significance of the endpoint, since the magnitude of the benefit is clear. Often this is the case.

Example: Psoriasis Area and Severity Index (PASI)

PASI is a complicated endpoint. It requires 20 measurements, with multiple calculations required. PASI is also ambiguous in some ways. For example, it requires judgement on the part of the physician on exactly where arms and legs begin, in order to calculate the amount of surface area impacted by the disease. It is also incomplete, in that it doesn't include itching and other factors that are important in the burden of disease. Finally, it is subjective, in that the percent of surface area involved is to a large degree subjective.

Unfortunately, for a pleimorphic disease, such as SLE, even remission can be difficult to define, since coming up with an endpoint that represents the entirety of a disease, but is at the same time quantifiable, can be difficult.

For composite endpoints, it is also important to insure that all negative outcomes are captured as part of the endpoint. For example, in a trial of severe congestive heart failure patients, a composite endpoint or even a non-composite one, would have to make allowances for death – if everyone dies, then the rate of recurrences would likely be very low (survival bias).

2.2 Example: Mean Value

Let's take one common endpoint to illustrate clinical relevance: the mean. In general, when we compare the mean measurement (for example, blood pressure) pre and post treatment, the underlying assumption is that the shape of the distribution curve doesn't change.

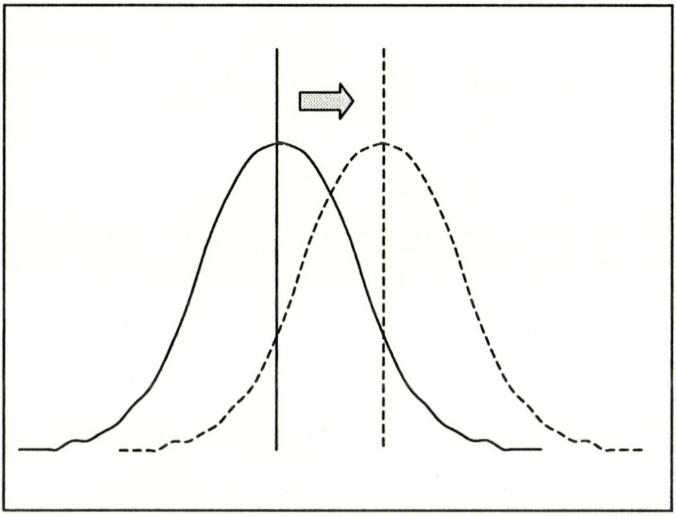

However, this is not necessarily true. In fact, many drugs only show a response in a subgroup of patients, as thus:

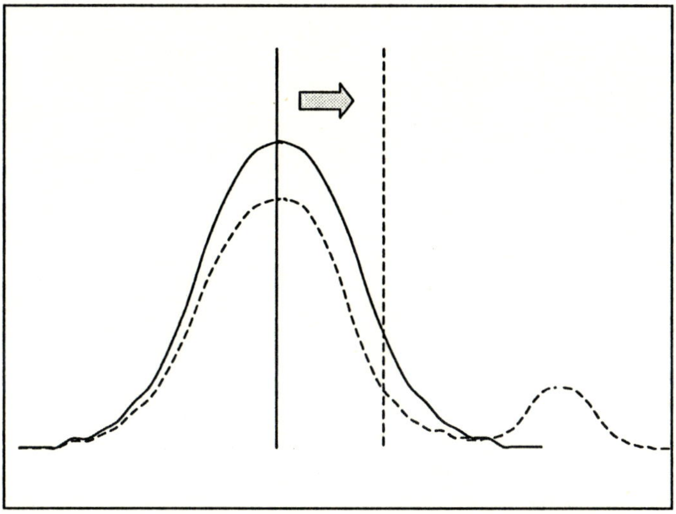

Or even worse, even if the mean improves, some patients may do worse.

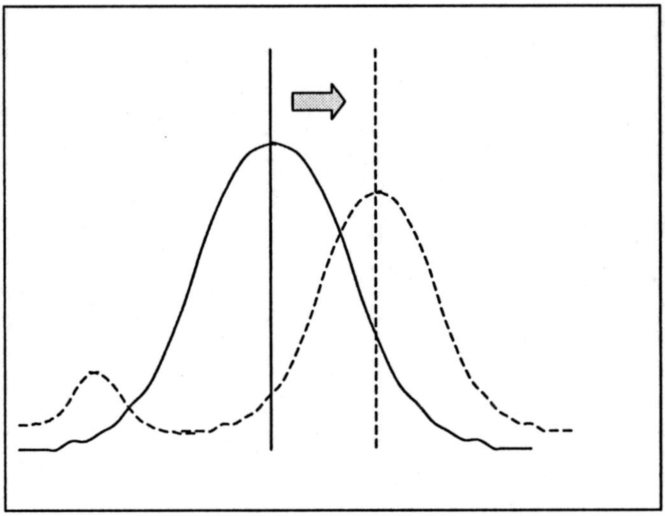

Or the mean might not change much but a subgroup might benefit.

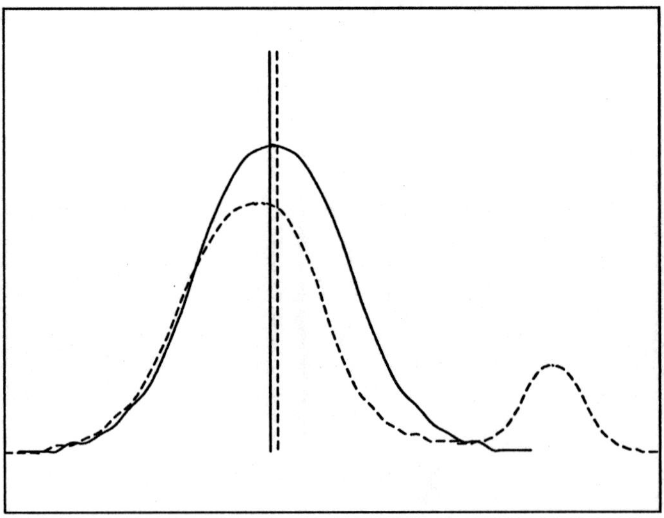

Depending on whether the subgroup can be predefined, and whether it's the same subgroup of patient who benefit, the drug may have utility even if it is not beneficial for the group as a whole.

Because of these considerations, and because each disease and each therapy acts differently, the choice of endpoints must be made carefully. Different situations might call for different endpoints such as: change in mean, number of patients who cross a certain threshold, subgroup analysis, etc.

In addition, there are multiple other dimensions of clinical response, such as durability of effect, time to onset of action, and tachyphlaxis, some of which can be captured in one endpoint but often need to be described separately.

2.3 Types of Endpoints

In addition, depending on the type of disease, the choice of endpoints that are clinically relevant can be different.

For an acute or subacute self-limiting disease, such as a cold, the appropriate endpoint generally relate to symptom reduction or decrease in the course of the disease, since the outcome is always a spontaneous cure.

For a disease that is not self-limiting, the ultimate outcome may be an appropriate endpoint, such as mortality. Increase in the length of time before the ultimate outcome such as time to death or time to disability may also be inappropriate. A disease with a significant burden of illness, symptom reduction such as decrease in pain may be an appropriate endpoint as well.

For a recurring disease with a waxing and waning course, induction of remission, increase in time between flares, or reduction in the frequencies of flares might all be clinically meaningful.

For vaccination studies, prevention of disease would be an appropriate endpoint.

Other considerations in clinical relevance of the endpoint include the length of response, and that can sometimes be an endpoint as well.

3 Responsiveness/Analysis

3.1 Background

Responsiveness is a critical characteristic of a good endpoint. The endpoint should be sensitive to changes in the clinical phenomenon being measured: when there is a change in the phenomenon, the value of the endpoint should change a well. Endpoints with good responsiveness allow smaller sample sizes and permit better estimate of the clinical benefit.

Of course, an extremely sensitive endpoint has the potential to detect even changes that may not be clinically significant, such as a 3% decrease in tumor size or 6 hr increased in median survival. It is important then to balance the responsiveness with clinical significance. For a pivotal Phase III study, the endpoint that is both responsive and clinically significant should be chosen for the primary endpoint.

Of course, in order to enable appropriate the risk benefit assessment, the trial should include secondary endpoints that are very responsive, in order to estimate the magnitude of the benefit. For Phase I or II, highly sensitive endpoint, even if it detects non-clinically significant changes, may be preferred so long as it is predictive of the Phase III endpoint.

In addition to the sensitivity of the measure, which is driven largely by the type of variable chosen, the other major factor in the responsiveness of the endpoint is the type of analysis applied to the endpoint.

What Determines an Endpoint's Responsiveness?

- Sensitivity of the measure (driven by type of variable: continuous, dichotomous, etc.)
- Type of analysis (mean change, survival, etc.)
- Susceptibility to treatment
- Length of follow-up
- Robustness to drop-outs

Below are the main types of analysis that can be performed. It is necessary to prespecify the analysis to be performed during the design phase, before study initiation, because it will determine the power of the study. It will also insure the research question being asked is specific. Also, prespecifying the endpoint and the analysis will satisfy the single hypothesis-testing criteria, in order to satisfy the convention for establishing causal relationship between the intervention and outcome. In theory, the primary endpoint and the analysis plan can be changed at any time before the unblinding, but this is considered poor form and might raise the suspicion of faulty blinding.

3.2 Landmark Analysis

Landmark analysis is measurement of an endpoint at a fixed time. Some examples are number of subjects alive 30 days after a myocardial infarction, or number of patients who are in remission 12 weeks after starting a therapy for Crohn's disease. This type of analysis is simple, and any variable – quantitative or qualitative – can be used with a landmark analysis. Imputation of missing values is also usually uncomplicated. For example, the proportion of patients with healed wounds at 8 weeks would be a landmark analysis, as would average percentage of area healed at 8 weeks.

One important drawback to landmark analysis is that it requires larger (often significantly larger) sample size than some of the other types of analysis. More importantly, landmark analysis is not suitable for certain clinical trials. For example, some diseases almost always resolve, and the drug might be intended to shorten the duration of disease, such as varicella.

The clinical utility of the drug might not be captured with a simple landmark analysis for diseases where duration of disease is important. In other diseases, such as lupus or multiple sclerosis, a study might be designed to reduce the likelihood of flares (or duration or severity of flares) and a landmark analysis may not be the most sensitive way to detect the clinical efficacy of the drug. This is because flares that occur and resolve before the landmark analysis would be ignored in the analysis.

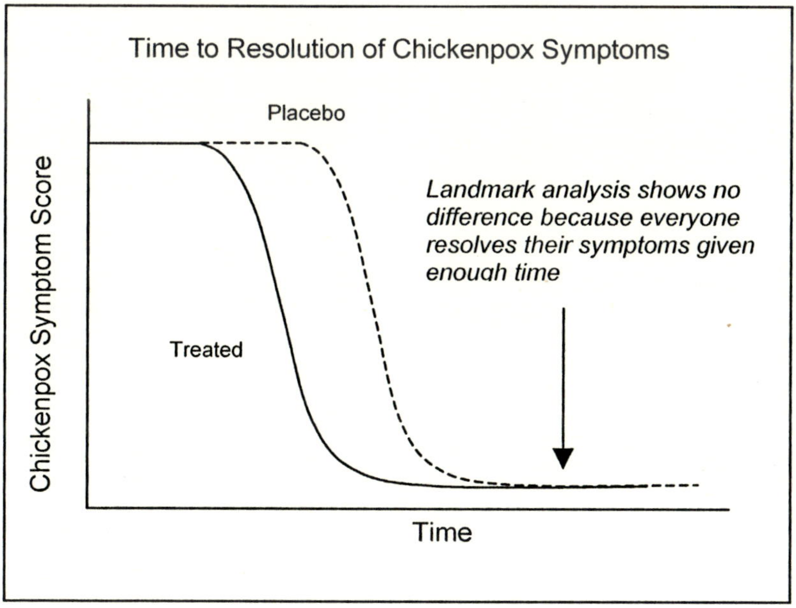

3.2.1 Unpaired Analysis

Landmark analysis can be done either solely on the post-treatment value or as pairwise comparison of pretreatment and post-treatment values (also called a change score). An example of unpaired analysis would be comparison of the mean height at 1 year in the placebo group *vs.* the growth hormone group at 1 year. If the initial value at randomization is fairly homogeneous, then unpaired analysis is reasonable.

3.2.2 Paired Analysis/Change Analysis

Change analysis or pairwise comparisons are often more sensitive than an unpaired analysis. An example of change analysis would be to compare the average growth (height at 1 year minus height pretreatment) between placebo and growth hormone. Or as another example, one might measure the average area of the remaining wound in a wound healing study, or calculate the percent decrease in the wound area. It should be noted that in this type of analysis, the difference in the pretreatment and post-treatment value in each patient is derived first, then the mean is calculated for each group (as opposed to deriving the average growth from subtracting mean pretreatment height from mean post-treatment height - this would result in loss of all individual data and weaken the analysis).

Change score is usually more powerful technique than an unpaired analysis, especially if the population is heterogeneous to being with – for example if the size of the wound varies significantly from 1 cm2 to 10 cm2. The sample size can often be substantially reduced with pairwise analysis.

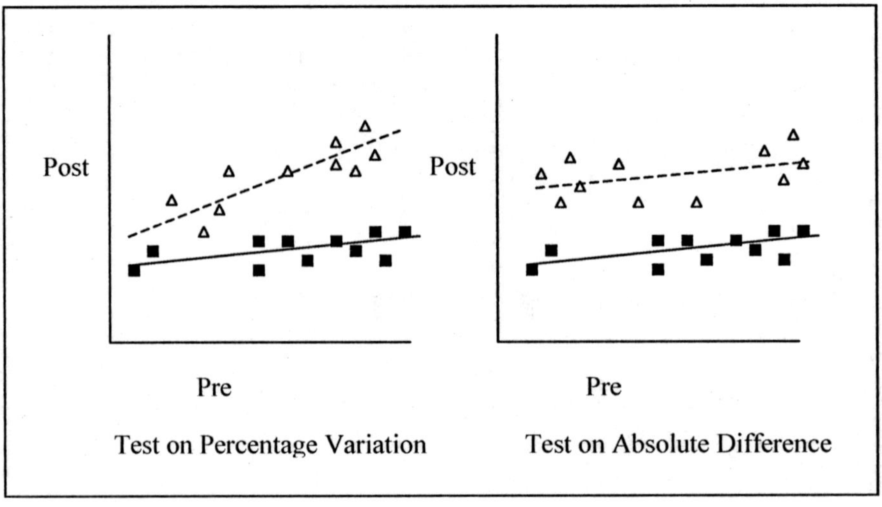

Also, when a change analysis is being performed, there is a choice to compare absolute difference or relative difference. For example, in a 60 cm child, the growth change can be expressed as 3 cm absolute growth or 5% relative growth. In general, most biological parameters will change as a percentage – for example, 20% improvement in joint count, or PASI-50 improvement in psoriasis. In those cases, percent difference is the appropriate change to compare.

If the difference is more clinical meaningful on an absolute basis or if the drug works similarly regardless of pretreatment value, then using absolute difference is reasonable

3.3 Frequency Analysis

For a disease with multiple recurrences such as SLE or asthma, measuring the frequency of flares can be an appropriate analysis. Since one patient can have more than one event, statistical power increases significantly.

However, several important caveats exist. First, the events should ideally be independent. That is, if the likelihood of having a subsequent flare increases after one flare, the analysis can become difficult, and more importantly, the increase in statistical power may not be realized. Second, it can sometimes be difficult to keep the patient in the trial after one or two flares, and imputation for patients who drop out can be a major challenge. In this type of trial, the dropouts almost certainly represent the sickest patients. Ignoring or censoring dropouts almost certainly introduce bias, but imputing an acceptable number of exacerbations for the patients can be difficult.

If the events are not independent, there are some techniques for analyzing the data. For instance, patients can be categorized into having no event, 1 event, 2 events, etc. This type of analysis does not require assuming independence of events, and though not as powerful as a frequency analysis, it is more powerful than simply dichotomizing the response into event/no event. There are also techniques that take into account the amount of independence among the events, but these techniques require some additional statistical assumptions and can be more complicated.

3.4 Repeated Measure Analysis/Slope Analysis

In some studies, a variable is measured multiple times over the course of the study – for example, blood pressure, visual acuity, glomerular filtration rate, etc. This is true particularly for a disease that is progressive or for a drug that has progressively better effects.

Often in clinical trials of this type, only the first and last measurements are used for analysis (the difference pre and post treatment with the drug is calculated). In effect, all the data collected in the middle are discarded. This is often because analyzing repeated measures data requires difficult statistical calculations, particularly with regard to missing data, and the possibility that biological and clinical response to the drug may be nonlinear.

However, for Phase II studies in particular, where sample sizes are smaller and less conservative statistical techniques are acceptable, multiple measures analysis is underutilized. If a biological phenomenon is known to have a linear progression, such as loss of glomerular filtration rate in polycystic kidney disease, slope of decline can be used, which is relatively straightforward statistical analysis. This is a much more powerful technique than just using pre and post differences in the outcome in that the variability can be significantly reduced. Also, it is easy to impute missing values – even if a patient drops out or they miss a visit, the slope can be calculated.

Similarly, if a drug improved FEV_1 gradually and progressively over time, comparing the slope can be a powerful way of measuring drug effect.

Also, sustained response – response at multiple endpoints is a variation on repeated measures, and is helpful in cases of high placebo rate. For instance, defining an endpoint as remission at week 10 and at week 12 for a Crohn's disease drug may increase the likelihood of a positive result, because it may decrease the rate of false remission in the placebo group.

If the change in the endpoint is non-linear, it is still possible to model the change over time and gain statistical power, but the shape of the curve must be known or at least a reasonable approximation must be known. Repeated measures analysis can be used to compare multiple measures. Alternatively, area under the cure method may be used to make use of multiple measures.

In general, repeat measures analysis can be very useful if the disease is waxing and waning. However, power may sometimes be decreased if such an analysis is used for a steadily progressive disease. In some cases, using just the last measurement may be more sensitive, because the difference in value between the treatment groups may be the most pronounced at later measurements. The impact on power is determined by the variability and the magnitude of the difference between the two groups over time. Low variability and a large difference in the treatment groups that increases over time makes repeat measures analysis less valuable.

3.5 Time-to-Event Analysis

For a drug designed to shorten the duration of a disease or a flare, such as a drug for varicella or for acute exacerbation of Crohn's disease, time-to-event analysis can be useful. Similarly, for drugs designed to improve survival or lengthen the time to recurrence of a disease, time-to-event analysis can be useful.

Time-to-event analysis, however, generally can be used for an endpoint that can only happen once, such as death. For events that can occur multiple times, time-to-first event can be used instead, such as time-to-first recurrence of atrial fibrillation.

Hazard Ratio

The actual analysis used in time-to-event analysis is, however, usually not time-to-event but a hazards ratio analysis. In an ideal situation, we would follow all patients until they experience the event. However, this is usually not practical due to time constraints, patient dropouts, and the fact that not every patient might have the event. The analysis is therefore performed with a hazard model – a statistical method of looking at the events that happen over time in the two groups.

As an aside, it is inappropriate to use mean time-to-event instead of a hazard model. For example, if in the placebo group 2 pts healed after 2 weeks and none thereafter, and in the treated group 2 healed at 2 weeks and 4 more at 6 weeks, average time to healing would be shorter in the placebo group.

Another advantage of a time-to-event analysis is that if the event rate is not known prior to the study, it is possible to specify the duration of follow-up in terms of number of events. For example, in oncology trials, the trial might run until a prespecified number of events have occurred.

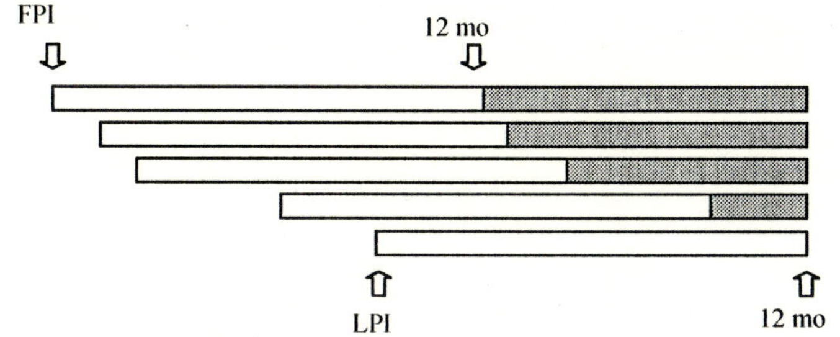

With survival analysis, the shaded periods can still contribute data, whereas in landmark analysis, only the white part can.

In addition, time-to-event or hazard analysis allows full use of all data from patients even if they had different lengths of follow-up. For studies that are difficult to enroll, hazard analysis allows the use of all the data.

So for example, for an multiple sclerosis study, if enrollment lasted 1 year and a minimum of 1 year of follow-up was required, then the first enrolled patient could have had 2 years of follow-up by the time last patient completed the 1 year follow-up. With landmark analysis, that first patient's second year would not contribute information to the primary endpoint at all, whereas with a hazard analysis, all the data could be used.

A caveat about hazard analysis is that usually, we must make the assumption is that the hazard ratio is constant over time. However, there are some clinical situations where the hazards cross. A classic paper illustrative of this was the prospective (though nonrandomized) study of transplantation *vs.* chemotherapy post induction of remission in AML.[1] In that study, the transplantation group fared worse in the first 6 months, but at 5 years, 49% of the patients in the group survived, compared to 20% of the control group.

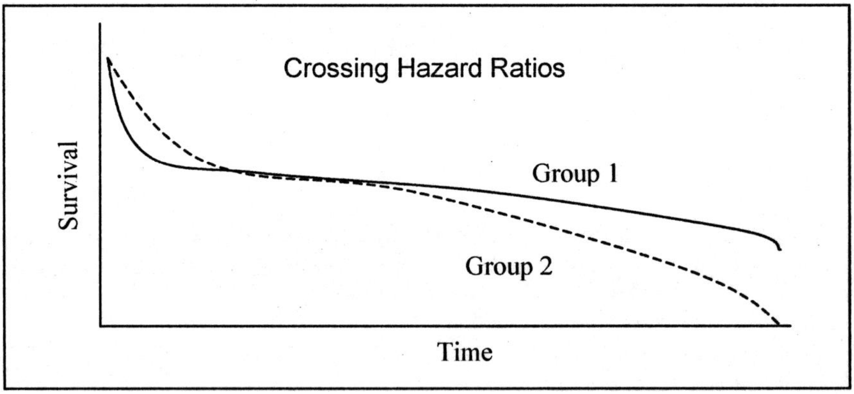

3.6 Susceptibility to Treatment

Another important factor in responsiveness is susceptibility to the treatment or intervention. For example, anti-IgE antibody would, by its mechanism of action, be expected to decrease exacerbations but not FEV_1. Similarly, a reperfusion injury protectant may be expected to protect against moderate or large CK-MB increases but not small leaks that are due to the trauma of the surgery itself (incisions, stitching, etc.)

Case Study: Pexelizumab in CABG

Pexelizumab was studied in a double-blind, randomized, placebo-controlled Phase II trial. Total of 914 patients were enrolled, with stratification into two groups: those undergoing only CABG or those undergoing CABG with concomitant valve surgery. Patients were treated with placebo, pexelizumab 2 mg/kg bolus, or pexelizumab 2 mg/kg bolus followed by a 24 hour infusion of pexelizumab at 0.05 mg/kg/hr.

The primary endpoint was 30 day composite of one or more of the following:

- Non-Q-wave myocardial infarction (NQWMI) defined as CK-MB elevation (mild, moderate, or severe)
- Neurological deficits
- Left ventricular dysfunction

The primary endpoint was obviously designed to maximize the event rate so that the sample size could be reduced. It was probably expected that NQWMI was going to drive the events.

The study missed the primary endpoint, which is not surprising given that multiple prior studies had shown that small CKMB leaks were due to the surgical procedure itself and not modifiable. An exploratory endpoint of moderate/severe NQWMI (CK-MB >100 ng/ml) or death was highly significant.

In this example, trying to increase the event rate by including broad range of outcome, in disregard of pathophysiology and prior clinical study results, led to a negative study.

4 Primary and Secondary Endpoints

4.1 Primary Endpoint

Primary endpoint occupies a special place in clinical trials. Primary endpoint is accepted to be the central hypothesis of a study, and a positive result on the primary endpoint is accepted as being sufficient to establish a causal relationship between the intervention and outcome. This is generally not true of other endpoints, although the convention is less clear in the case of a positive primary endpoint and concurrent results in related outcomes. Certainly, if the primary endpoint not being met, no other endpoint can be held to be establishing a causal relationship.

For Phase III or pivotal studies, there generally is one prespecified primary endpoint with an alpha of 0.05. The endpoint is usually an efficacy endpoint. This is the accepted standard for a "positive" study, with the thought that if a study yields results that are not likely to occur more than 5% of the time by chance, it is sufficiently compelling to be accepted as being true.

The p value of 0.05 is arbitrary and has been accepted traditionally as the bar for a positive study—for establishing causality. The p value represents the likelihood of having the results by chance. So p value of 0.05 indicates that the results could have been seen by chance 5% of the time. Or to state it another way, if the same trial were performed infinite number of times, and if the drug had absolutely no efficacy, similar or more convincing result would be seen about 1 time out of 20.

Also, as discussed in a separate section, p values is not as informative as the confidence interval, and because of this the confidence interval is becoming a more common standard in interpretation of study results.

Regulatory Point: Reproducibility of Studies and p Value

In general, FDA requires two studies with a p value of 0.05 or less (two sided). The reasons for it are multiple, but the main reason is to increase confidence in the validity of the study results. They want reproducibility, to make sure it wasn't a fluke, that it wasn't due to some special aspect of the study (certain sites, the batch of drug, etc.), and to avoid fraud. Also, they want to improve the validity of the study by insuring that in a slightly different population or slightly different endpoint that the drug works as well – in this way, they add to the confidence in convergent validity.

This requirement was put into place by CDER a while ago when the studies were not as robust. Now that the studies in general are well designed, double blind, placebo-controlled studies, there is argument that there is less need for this. Furthermore, the FDA has stated that a single study can be acceptable for approval if it is robust. By this, they mean:

- $P<0.00125$ (0.05 x 0.05 divided by 2)
- Internal consistency across subgroups
- Internal consistency across endpoints

It should be noted that in very large trials (e.g., 17,000 patient thrombolytic trial), trials with very clear results (mortality endpoint and low p value), trials that would be unethical or repeat, or for CBER products, FDA has not been as strict with the requirement for two trials.

4.2 Co-Primary Endpoints

By convention, one study can test only one primary endpoint at alpha of 0.05, unless it is a factorial study.

The only common exception to this is in the case of multi-armed studies where several different therapies are being compared against the same control arm or in dose ranging studies. In those cases, although the most rigorous analysis would require correction for multiple comparisons, in practice the corrections may not be made. Strictly speaking, this is not quite appropriate.

Also for indications such as sepsis where nearly 30 negative studies were performed with various therapeutics before activated protein C show efficacy, it would be reasonable to think about correcting for multiple number of times trials were conducted, but this is generally not done.

However, there are instances where it is necessary or desirable to answer multiple causal questions. In such a case there are some limited options, as below.

4.2.1 Splitting the Alpha

For multiple primary endpoints, it is permissible to split the alpha – require for example if there are two primary endpoints that the significance be established with a p value of less than 0.025. If either one meets p value of 0.025 then a causal relationship is inferred. Any combination of primary endpoints with p of .05 would be acceptable: .04 + 0.01; 0.01 + 0.01 + 0.01 + 0.01 + 0.01; etc.

In fact, in theory, if the primary endpoint were that both co-primary endpoints had to be met, then each endpoint meeting p value of 0.22 should suffice (0.22 x 0.22 = 0.05), but it would be very unconventional to propose something like that.

4.2.2 Hierarchical Testing

Alternatively, hierarchical testing (sometimes also referred to as use of contingent primary endpoints) is performed. This can be for subgroups or for endpoint. For example, if the drug meets p value of 0.05 for the overall group, then a subgroup can be tested with p value of 0.05 as the standard for establishing significance. If multiple subgroups are examined, then it is appropriate to correct for multiple comparisons.

Similarly, if the study is shown to be non-inferior, then superiority may be tested with p-value of 0.05. Or, if an endpoint of death/disability is met, then a second hierarchical test for disability alone may be performed.

In each of these cases, the second test is a sub-question of the primary question. The second test cannot be performed if the first is negative. This is intuitive for the noninferiority. Obviously, it is not possible for a drug to be equivalent if it is inferior. It is less intuitive for subgroups – obviously it is possible for a drug to be efficacious in a subgroup and not for the group as a whole. For example, Herceptin works only for breast cancer patients with HER2 overexpression. The reason for this is discussed in more detail in the subgroup section below, but essentially, it is to avoid multiple comparisons that can lead to a spurious result. It is not that a drug may not work for a subgroup – it is that the trial cannot be used as evidence for that conclusion.

Another way to putting it is that if both endpoints must be met in order for the results to be considered positive, hierarchical testing is appropriate and alpha does not need to be split.

4.3 Secondary Endpoints

Prespecified secondary endpoints are used for many different purposes, including:

- Examine pharmacokinetic and pharmacodynamic
- Examine important safety parameters
- Examine non-clinical endpoints
- Examine alternate ways of evaluating the primary endpoint
- Examine pharmacoeconomic results
- Examine resource utilization
- Examine quality of care outcome

Often, the secondary endpoints are used in an undisciplined fashion to examine a plethora of issues. In general, the number of secondary endpoints should be as few as possible, because a large number of secondary endpoints increase the likelihood of both Type I and Type II errors. Given enough secondary endpoints, a spurious negative result is likely—for example, a subgroup may appear not to benefit—and a spurious positive result is almost certain. Secondary endpoints should be carefully selected to examine clinically meaningful questions that are not replicates of each other.

Secondary endpoints do serve an important role in quantifying the magnitude of benefit, and in examining important safety and clinical utility parameters.

Even if the trial is positive, in that the primary efficacy endpoint is met, the ultimate utility of the therapy is dependent on a risk-benefit analysis. While the result of the primary endpoint is usually dichotomized into positive/negative ($p<0.05$ or $p=>0.05$), the amount of clinical efficacy is important in determining the risk/benefit. A sensitive secondary endpoint that can estimate the degree of benefit can be very helpful, as can estimates of pharmacoeconomic or quality of life benefit.

In addition, factors such as time to response, relapse/durability of response, rebound, tachyphlaxis, can and often should be examined as secondary endpoints.

5 Composite Endpoints

5.1 Background

Composite endpoint is an endpoint made up of several parameters, such as ACR20 score or PASI score. This is in comparison to a simple endpoint such as death or FEV_1.

In general, a simple endpoint is preferred because composite endpoints, by their very nature, are prone to bias and makes interpretation more difficult. At a minimum, it makes the analysis of the result an approximation of a continuous, variable, and therefore makes the interpretation an approximation. No composite endpoint is truly linear.

Caveat:

It should be noted that a non-composite endpoint is not necessarily immune to some of some of the issues associated with composite endpoints, se issues. There may be heterogeneity with those endpoints as well. Fore example, fracture is a simple endpoint, but vertebral fractures may be different in pathophysiology, response to drug, and clinical significance from wrist fractures. Similarly, 10% skin involvement of atopic dermatitis may be very different in clinical significance if it's on the face *vs.* on the trunk.

Also, individual components of a composite endpoint may sometimes go in opposite directions, which makes such a result extremely difficult to interpret. However, there are instances where composite endpoints are necessary or appropriate. They include the following.

Low Event Rate – Increase Sensitivity:

Sometimes a trial is not feasible because the sample size would be too large unless a composite endpoint is used. Thrombolytic trials, for example, require over 20,000 patients because the current mortality rate is 5%.

Also, in Phase II studies, a composite endpoint might make a reasonable sized trial feasible.

A major caveat in designing composite endpoint to increase the event rate is that the individual endpoints must be sensitive to the treatment effect. If they are not, then it dilutes the effect of the drug. Also, the additional endpoint should not be a competing risk. For example, the endpoint of death/congestive heart failure may be a worse endpoint than death alone, even if the overall rate is higher, because if reduction in death might increase the number of patients with congestive heart failure (those who would have died live but live with congestive heart failure).

Difficult-to-Diagnose – Increase Specificity:

For some diseases, the endpoint is nonspecific, and several clinical manifestations may be required before an event can be clearly classified as a clinical event driven by the disease. For example, to qualify as a true exacerbation of multiple sclerosis, one might require MRI finding in addition to clinical findings or clinical finding of a certain severity or duration.

This should be compared with using a subset of events as the endpoint, which is technically refining an endpoint and not subject to some of the issues associated with composite endpoints (for example, anterior myocardial infarction is a subset of myocardial infarction's, not a composite – just because an endpoint has to meet multiple criteria doesn't necessarily make it a composite endpoint.) This is a semantic distinction. Conceptually, a subset of events and composite endpoint designed to increase specificity are the same—requiring that the endpoint meet multiple criteria.

Heterogeneity:

In some instances, there is heterogeneity in the presentation of the disease, and in order to fully capture the clinical significance of the disease, a composite endpoint in necessary. This can be due to several different factors:

Pleiotropic Disease:

Some diseases, such as lupus have protean manifestations, and the only way to capture the true severity of the disease is to have a composite endpoint. Otherwise a score might improve when a patient get worse.

Changes in the Course of the Disease:

Some diseases change their manifestations over time such that it would be difficult to have a uniform measure of severity. For example, for MS, time to walk a certain distance may be appropriate at certain stage, but not after the disease has progressed beyond a certain point.

Heterogeneous Population:

Some diseases might have subpopulations that manifest their disease in different ways. Often it may be better to examine the population in separate studies but it may not be possible to do that.

Dropouts:

In some instances, where dropouts, crossovers, or rescue medications are expected, a composite endpoint that includes dropouts as an event may be appropriate

Avoid Survivor Bias/Competing Risk:

Sometimes it is necessary to include the more severe potential outcomes even if the primary effect is expected to occur on another outcome. For example, if the drug is expected to have little effect on mortality and significant effect on congestive heart failure hospitalization, but the patient population is at risk for death, it may be necessary to include death in order to avoid survivor bias. Otherwise, it may turn out that the drug kills patients who would have been merely hospitalized, and hospitalizations decrease because the sickest patients have died.

Capture Efficacy and Safety in Same Endpoint:

Sometimes, a drug will have a serious adverse effect. Or, the comparator drug may have a serious side effect that the new drug is not expected to have. In those cases, a composite endpoint that encompasses efficacy and safety may be appropriate. An example is net clinical benefit endpoint composed of death/intracranial hemorrhage after thrombolytic therapy.

5.2 Types of Composite Endpoints

Unweighted Composite Endpoints with Alternate/Exclusive/Independent Events:

As was previously mentioned, composite endpoints are commonly used when the simple endpoint in occurs infrequent, such as in acute coronary syndrome trials. For GP IIb/IIIa trials, composite of death/myocardial infarction/refractory ischemia has been used.

These endpoints typically are alternate independent events: for example, an endpoint might specify "event A *or* event B *or* event C."

An endpoint such as this is problematic at best for several reasons.

- It asserts that a death is similar in clinical significance as an episode of recurrent ischemia
- It suggests that the three types of events are biologically related. This is because these events have been selected together and not other endpoints or safety endpoints suggesting that there is a biological rationale for combining these and not other endpoints.

As previously noted, an endpoint can combine efficacy and safety endpoints. For example, death of intracranial hemorrhage is a traditional endpoint in thrombolytic trials.

A composite endpoint that has alternate events is usually dichotomous. However, if each event is exclusive, a count variable can be formulated. For example, an endpoint might be: total number of myocardial infarction's, strokes, PTCA's and CABG's. This type of a composite event still suffers from the issue of asserting each event is equal in clinical significance as the others.

Weighted Composite Endpoints with Exclusive Events:

One way of addressing the issue of the fact that different events have different clinical significance is by weighting the endpoints – so for example, death might be given a score of 5, Mi score of 3 and recurrent ischemia a score of 2.

Similar scoring system is found in diseases such as Lupus, where some of the composite scores are weighted average of the various endpoints (see SLEDAI example).

Weighted endpoints can sometimes approximate a continuous or count variables, and are added, subtracted, etc., but this is problematic in that one point from one type of event (cerebritis) is not necessarily the same as one point from another type of event (urinary cast). It is necessary to assert that each point on the scoring scale is identical or very similar in clinical significance no matter which endpoint was responsible for the point. The most clinically meaningful way to treat them is by dichotomizing or categorizing them. For example, score below 50 on a score may be considered remission, score above 100 considered a flare, etc.

Ideally, the events would also be exclusive and independent of each other, because otherwise the scoring becomes very complicated. For example, someone who dies cannot have further events so death is not independent of any other event. It would be difficult to assign a score to death in any scoring system.

An additional issue is that it is sometimes difficult to gain consensus on the appropriate weighting of the various endpoints.

Non-Weighted Composite Ordinal Endpoints:

Alternate type of composite endpoint is a non-weighted endpoint, such ACR20. These endpoints are at best ordinal. Often they specify that certain combination of factors be satisfied in order to qualify as an event or to qualify for a score.

ACR scores are good examples of scores that appears to be quantitative but is actually ordinal at best. ACR20 is not 20% improvement in rheumatoid arthritis. It is a complex composite, requiring at least 20% improvement on several parameters, which must include both tender joint count and swollen joint count, and 3 out 5 other parameters. Similarly, ACR50 requires 50% improvement on multiple parameters, and ACR70 requires 70%, etc.

One of the goals for ACR20 is to have high specificity for improvement, which requires multiple separate improvement outcomes. ACR20 is specific and sensitive in determining improvement in individual patients, but it is not a continuous measure. ACR 70% is not 20% better than ACR50, and ACR50 is not 2.5 times better than ACR20.

ACR is not a continuous endpoint

In order to achieve ACR50, the patient must have 50% improvement in multiple parameters, which is usually much more difficult than achieving 50% mean improvement. Even if the patient has a dramatic improvement in one or two components, the response must be consistent across multiple parameters. The difference between 50% and 20% minimal improvement on multiple parameters is much more difficult than difference between mean 20% and 50% improvements.

ACR is not a true ordinal endpoint:

Also, although in general a patient with ACR70 will have had a clinically better response than a patient with ACR20 or ACR50 response, this is not necessarily true. A patient who has 90% improvement in 6 out 7 parameters except tender joint count which improved 20% will have ACR20 response while a patient who had 50% improvement in 5 out of 7 parameters could have ACR50 response. So in fact, ACR score is an approximation of an ordinal endpoint but is actually nominal. In practice, ACR scores approximate an ordinal endpoint closely enough that it is often treated as one.

<table>
<tr><th colspan="2">ACR 20 Definition of Improvement in Rheumatoid Arthritis</th></tr>
<tr><th>Both of the below criteria must be met</th><th>3 out of the below 5 criteria must improve by ≥ 20%</th></tr>
<tr><td rowspan="3">1. ≥ 20% improvement in tender joint count</td><td>1. Patient pain assessment</td></tr>
<tr><td>2. Patient global assessment</td></tr>
<tr><td>3. Physician global assessment</td></tr>
<tr><td rowspan="2">2. ≥ 20%improvement in swollen joint count</td><td>4. Patient self-assessed disability</td></tr>
<tr><td>5. Acute-phase reactant (ESR or CRP)</td></tr>
</table>

Systemic Lupus Erythematous Disease Activity Index (SLEDAI) Score Endpoint

Each sign or symptom is given a weighted score, and the sum of the scores is the SEDAI score.

Score	Definition
8	Seizure Recent onset. Exclude metabolic, infectious, drug causes.
8	Psychosis Altered ability to function in normal activity due to severe disturbance in the perception of reality. Include hallucinations, incoherence, marked loose associations, impoverished thought content, marked illogical thinking, bizarre, disorganized, or catatonic behavior. Exclude uremia and drug causes.
8	Organic brain syndrome Altered mental function with impaired orientation, memory, or other intellectual function, with rapid onset and fluctuating clinical features. Include clouding of consciousness with reduced capacity to focus, and inability to sustain attention to environment, plus at least 2 of the following: perceptual disturbance, incoherent speech, insomnia or daytime drowsiness, or increased or decreased psychomotor activity. Exclude metabolic, infectious, or drug causes.
8	Visual disturbance Retinal changes of SLE. Include cytoid bodies, retinal hemorrhages, serous exudate or hemorrhages in the choroid, or optic neuritis. Exclude hypertension, infection, or drug causes.
8	Cranial nerve disorder New onset of sensory or motor neuropathy involving cranial nerves.
8	Lupus headache Severe, persistent headache; may be migrainous, but must be nonresponsive to narcotic analgesia.
8	CVA New onset of cerebrovascular accident(s). Exclude arteriosclerosis.
8	Vasculitis Ulceration, gangrene, tender finger nodules, periungual infarction, splinter hemorrhages, or biopsy or angiogram proof of vasculitis.
4	Arthritis More than 2 joints with pain and signs of inflammation (i.e., tenderness, swelling, or effusion).
4	Myositis Proximal muscle aching/weakness, associated with elevated creatine phosphokinase/aldolase or electromyogram changes or a biopsy showing myositis.
4	Urinary casts Heme-granular or red blood cell casts.
4	Hematuria > 5 red blood cells/high power field. Exclude stone, infection, or other cause.
4	Proteinuria > 0.5 gm/24 hours. New onset or recent increase of more than 0.5 gm/24 hours.
4	Pyuria > 5 white blood cells/high power field. Exclude infection.
2	New rash New onset or recurrence of inflammatory type rash.
2	Alopecia New onset or recurrence of abnormal, patchy or diffuse loss of hair.
2	Mucosal ulcers New onset or recurrence of oral or nasal ulcerations.
2	Pleurisy Pleuritic chest pain with pleural rub or effusion, or pleural thickening.
2	Pericarditis Pericardial pain with at least 1 of the following: rub, effusion, or electrocardiogram or echocardiogram confirmation.
2	Low complement Decrease in CH50, C3, or C4 below the lower limit of normal for testing laboratory.
2	Increased DNA binding > 25% binding by Farr assay or above normal range for testing laboratory.
1	Fever > 38°C. Exclude infectious cause.
1	Thrombocytopenia < 100,000 platelets/mm3.
1	Leukopenia < 3,000 white blood cells/mm3. Exclude drug causes.

Crohn's Disease Activity Index CDAI

CDAI = 2x1 + 5x2 + 7x3 + 20x4 + 30x5 + 10x6 + 6x7 + (weight factor)8

Crohn's disease activity index (CDAI) was meant originally to gauge the progress or lack of progress for people with Crohn's disease. However, since the original study, researchers have used it for broader purposes.

1. Number (total) of liquid or very soft stools in one week

2. Sum of seven daily abdominal pain ratings:
   (0=none, 1=mild, 2=moderate, 3=severe)

3. Sum of seven daily ratings of general well-being:
   (0=well, 1=slightly below par, 2=poor, 3=very poor, 4=terrible)

4. Symptoms or findings presumed related to Crohn's disease
   Add 1 for each set that corresponding to patient's symptoms:
   set 1: arthritis or arthralgia
   set 2: iritis or uveitis
   set 3: erythema nodosum, pyoderma gangrenosum, apththous stomatitis
   set 4: anal fissure, fistula or perirectal abscess
   set 5: other bowel-related fistula
   set 6: febrile (fever) episode over 100 degrees during past week.

5. Taking Lomotil or opiates for diarrhea
   0=no 1=yes

6. Abnormal mass
   0=none; 0.4=questionable; 1=present

7. Hematocrit [(Typical - Current) x 6]

8. 100 x [(standard weight-actual body weight) / standard weight]

Best WR, et al., "Development of a Crohn's disease activity index." Gastroenterology 70:439-444, 1976.

6 Safety Endpoints

6.1 Characteristics of Safety Endpoints

6.1.1 Relationship Between Efficacy and Safety Endpoints

At the first glance, efficacy and safety endpoints may seem to be opposite in a symmetrical fashion: safety seems to be equal and opposite of efficacy. In truth, these two types of endpoints are at best complements of each other—opposite but not equal—and different in profound and complicated ways.

All Endpoints can be Efficacy or Safety Endpoints

First of all, efficacy and safety endpoints are not two mutually exclusive sets of outcomes. That is to say, there is not a set of endpoints that are efficacy endpoints (survival, increase in time-to-event, remission) and another set of endpoints that are safety endpoints (death, bleeding, infection).

Depending on the context, and depending on the study, efficacy endpoints can be safety endpoints, and vice-versa. A key difference between efficacy and safety endpoints is the direction of change in the outcome. To put it another way, it is not so much that efficacy endpoints are one group of clinical endpoints and safety endpoints are another. Rather, efficacy endpoints are endpoints that change for the better; safety endpoints are ones that change for the worse.

For example, death can be an efficacy endpoint in one study and safety in another. If mortality rate decreases, it can be called survival benefit and be an efficacy endpoint. If it increases, it can be called fatality or serious adverse event and be a safety endpoint. Similarly, if asthma exacerbations increase, it can be a safety endpoint and if it decreases, it can be an efficacy endpoint.

Efficacy Needs Specificity; Safety Needs Sensitivity:

Also, the primary and secondary efficacy endpoints are normally prespecified, and the hypothesis being tested is usually the primary efficacy endpoint. Safety endpoints may or may not be prespecified. (Leaving aside for now the "safety studies" as well as the fact that most studies are two-tailed so that in effect most primary endpoints are both efficacy and safety endpoints)

The difference is that even an unexpected safety endpoint is treated as a valid clinical event, while unexpected efficacy events are generally treated as hypothesis generating. Also, a safety event or events do not need to reach significance in order to be considered a signal. To repeat, safety endpoints – changes in negative direction of a clinical endpoint – can be given credence even if non-prespecified and not statistically significant while the efficacy endpoints that are not prespecified are considered to be spurious. This is particularly true for major, severe adverse events. In this way, safety and efficacy endpoints are not reciprocal. This is because the tolerance for false positive result on efficacy is low and the specificity that is demanded is high; while the tolerance for false negative result on safety is low and high sensitivity for safety signal is important.

Characteristics of Safety Endpoints

Goes in negative direction (is detrimental to patient)
Not always prespecified
Not always validated
Not always randomized or stratified in advance
Not necessarily required to be statistically significant

The relationship between efficacy and safety is complementary in another aspect. Safety generally includes all clinically relevant, detrimental events not specified as an efficacy event. In other words, anything not specified as efficacy could be considered a safety endpoint. For example, if the primary efficacy endpoint is reduction in exacerbations of asthma, the safety endpoint could be everything else, such as hospitalizations or mortality. In this way, even if the efficacy endpoint is chosen carefully to maximize the likelihood of showing a benefit, the other clinically relevant endpoints can never be excluded completely from the outcome assessment, since they will be included in the safety analysis. For example, a drug that reduced asthma exacerbations but increased mortality would not be assessed on the basis of exacerbations alone.

In addition, unlike with most efficacy endpoints, the details of safety events can be important, and should be captured carefully in the clinical trial. Unlike efficacy, which almost always requires statistical analysis of aggregate data, even a single or a handful of safety events can be meaningfully analyzed in a descriptive fashion. For example, a single case of eosinophilia myalgia syndrome can be significant. A single case of highly unusual course of a common disease, in an atypical population, can also be meaningful. These types of dramatic events can occur with efficacy, but generally, such responses are often not a subject of a clinical trial, since if the conclusions from them are clear enough, and the bias from placebo effect and other confounders can be accounted for, a large scale randomized prospective clinical trial may not be needed.

6.1.2 Limitations of Safety Endpoints in Clinical Trials

The sample sizes for clinical trials are usually based on efficacy endpoints. The studies therefore are large enough and have enough power to detect only some of the adverse events, the ones that occur relatively frequently.

Even when trials are powered for specific rare adverse events, it is almost impossible to make them large enough to detect very rare events with any reliability. For example, even a trial with 30,000 patients would not be able to detect a very rare severe adverse event that occurred in 1 in 100,000 patients.

In addition, as was mentioned earlier, the constraints associated with efficacy endpoints, such as statistical significance, prespecification, and prohibition against multiple comparisons does not always apply to safety endpoints. This is because the bar for acknowledging safety events is much lower than for efficacy. So another limitation of safety endpoints in the reduction in rigor that is often unavoidable because it is not possible to predict, and therefore prespecify, in advance what all the potential safety issues may be.

However, for events that can be anticipated, a prospective safety analysis plan should be prepared. With such a plan, much stronger conclusions can be drawn since the events were prespecified. It also makes it less likely that a safety signal could be rationalized away or hidden by recategorizing events or analyzing the data in an inappropriate fashion.

6.1.3 Safety Endpoint Characteristics and Clinical Relevance

The broad categories of safety endpoints are discussed in following sections. However, the specific characteristics of safety events that can give it more or less clinical relevance. These are enumerated in this section.

Some safety endpoints are increase in an event of a risk that exists in the population at baseline. The risk of coronary events in osteoarthritis patients taking rofecoxib would be one example. These patients tend to have comorbidities and tend to have baseline risk factors for such events. These types of risks are more difficult to detect than the new risks that are generally not present such as arrhythmia and sudden death in young patients taking terfenadine. These patients are often otherwise healthy young women and tend to have no underlying risk factors for arrhythmias.

Some safety endpoints have harbinger or sentinel events. Others have indicators that allow early detection and intervention. For example, amaurosus fugax can be a harbinger for stroke, and nuisance gum bleeding can be a harbinger for intracranial bleeding. Events with a harbinger sign can be more easily detected in clinical trials than ones that cannot.

Reversible toxicities are much less worrisome than irreversible effects. Whether the toxicity is reversible or not has an enormous impact on clinical trial design and the use of the drug. Similarly, if the drug has an antidote or is dialyzable in an emergency, that has similar important implications.

If a toxicity has a harbinger sign or has a gradual onset of action – for example thrombocytopenia that develops over several weeks that reverse with withdrawal of drug, this is a very different type of toxicity than abrupt onset of agranulocytosis or a toxicity that is impossible to stop once it has started.

Certain safety events are reversible, such as asthma exacerbations and other are not, such as a stroke.

Some safety endpoints are treatable, such as an infection. And others have no treatment modality available.

With some safety endpoints, it is possible to screen patients at higher risk, whereas with other, this is not possible.

6.2 Clinical Trial Design Aspects

6.2.1 Anticipated Safety Events

Based on preclinical data and data from previous studies, and data from related compounds, it is often possible to anticipate certain safety events. For example, a new beta-blocker might be expected to have an effect on asthma. Anticipated safety events should be collected prospectively, and the events should be elicited. Each patient should be specifically asked about the specific type of event.

Some toxicities are intimately associated with the biological effect, are merely extensions of the desired biological effect. Examples include intracranial hemorrhage with thrombolytics and infections with immunosuppressive agents. In such cases, it might be impossible to dissociate the toxicity from the therapeutic effect. Indeed, for biologic agents, the most common toxicities are exactly this type.

Some toxicities are associated with the target, for example, renal toxicity with calcineurin inhibitors or protein kinase c effects with protein kinase c inhibitors (because it is hard to target one protein kinase c and not others). In other words, some biological process are closely linked by molecule phylogeny or pathophysiology and it is difficult to dissociate them. Some enzymes and molecules serve multiple processes, such as ADP or potassium channels – that is why antidiabetic drugs such as sulfonylureas decrease myocyte preconditioning, since both pancreatic cells and myocyte depend on potassium channels for physiological function.

The chemical structures also cause side effects, such as side chains associated with particular side effects such as QT prolongation and hepatotoxicity.

It's important keeping mind that sometimes the metabolites can cause toxicity, as can excipients, contaminants, and host cell proteins.

6.2.2 Harbinger Safety Events

In addition, for side effects that may not be a cause for alarm in and of itself, but may be harbingers of more rare and serious events, should be collected. Examples would include nuisance bleeding that might portend more serious bleeding in a few patients, mild thrombocytopenia that might portend severe thrombocytopenia in a subset of patients, and LFT abnormalities as harbinger of liver failure.

6.2.3 Unanticipated Safety Events

It is impossible to anticipate all possible safety events. The clinical study design and conduct must be such that unexpected safety events can be collected and analyzed. In addition to routine laboratory monitoring, there should be enough flexibility in the collection process to insure that unusual unanticipated events get captured.

There are, however, two broad categories of unanticipated safety events that should be captured in almost all trials. The first category includes events that are often seen with the particular type of intervention, in general. For small molecule drugs, these would include

- QT_c prolongation
- Liver toxicity
- Nephrotoxicity
- Bone marrow toxicity
- Drug-drug interaction

For biologics, they would include

- Immunogenicity
- Infusion reaction

The second broad category is severe, catastrophic safety events. These include death, malignancies, hospitalization, etc. Most of these are collected by the serious adverse event reporting system.

Rebound and tachyphlaxis are two types of adverse events that can occur with any drug. Both should be collected and characterized, either as efficacy or safety endpoints, since both are important in the way that the drug is used.

6.3 Safety Endpoint Collection Technique

6.3.1 Collection Frequency

The frequency of visits or data collection can increase the rate of events. This is because recall of events, especially minor events decreases over time, and after a week or so, minor adverse events are frequently forgotten.

6.3.2 Elicitation

Eliciting safety events, by specifically asking the patient whether he has experienced a safety event of this or that type will increase the frequency of the events. For example, if a patient is specifically asked whether he had a headache, he is more likely to recall it than if he were just asked if he experienced any adverse events.

6.3.3 Classification of Adverse Events

Safety events can be classified in a number of different ways. The severity is often graded mild, moderate, and severe.

Safety events can also be graded by regulatory definitions. FDA classifies events as serious or nonserious, and as expected or unexpected. The definitions are

6.3.4 Adverse Events *vs.* Disease Progression

In some cases, the disease progression may be difficult to distinguish from adverse event. An example would be death in an antiarrhythmic study. Sudden deaths in a population already at risk for arrhythmias post a myocardial infarction could be caused by congestive heart failure, arrhythmia, or proarrhythmia.

6.4 Special circumstances and Interactions with Other Factors

As was previously mentioned, some toxicities do not manifest until enough physiological damage has occurred to overcome the natural reserve of the organ system. In an analogous manner, some toxicities do not become apparent until the patients are in a physiologically stressful situation or are challenged. For example, tumor necrosis factor (tumor necrosis factor) inhibitors reactivate tuberculosis only in patients with pre-existing latent infections. Patients who have a negative PPD skin test would be unlikely to suffer reactivation of their tuberculosis. Other examples would be hypokalemia (digitalis, antiarrhythmics) unmasking proarrhythmic toxicities with antiarrhythmic drugs and infections unmasking adrenal insufficiency in patients on long-term systemic corticosteroids.

Some toxicities occur in a uniform fashion – essentially everyone who gets the drug experience the event. Other toxicities occur only in a subgroup of patients. For example, a particular subpopulation such as the elderly or certain ethnic groups may be a particularly high (or low) risk of experiencing adverse events in reaction to a drug.

Of the toxicities that occur in a subgroup, some occur randomly. For example, 10% of the patients might experience nausea each time the drug is administered, but different patients might experience it each time. Every patient has 10% chance of experiencing nausea each time they take the drug. This may be due to the way the drug works, or due to factors that can't be identified and are random, or to external factors that are beyond the control of the patients or physician.

Other toxicities occur in the same subgroup of patients – either because of underling genotype (metabolic enzyme allotypes, for example), phenotype/concomitant diseases (renal insufficiency, for example), or exposure to environmental factors (smoking, sunlight exposure, etc.). For example, the 10% of the patients with the highest tumor burden might experience chills during the drug infusion.

For the latter type of toxicities, if it is possible to identify in advance the population that is at risk, then the clinical trials and the risk-benefit of the drug can be modified. For either type, if the toxicities is gradual in onset and can be reversed upon discontinuation of the drug, then it is possible to monitor the patients early and avoid worst of the effects.

There are multiple other factors that can cause tremendous differences in the toxicity profile, such as differences in metabolism among patients; concomitant medications; concomitant diet (taking some medications on full stomach can alter absorption); non-concomitant diet (green vegetables that contain vitamin K may counteract some of the effects of coumadin, grapejuice can interfere with calcium channel blocker metabolism by impairing cytochrome P450 dependent metabolism); etc.

When designing a trial, it is important to take into account all these potential factors, and where appropriate, designing the trial or collecting data in an appropriate way. For example, for a platelet inhibitor that will be used frequently with anticoagulants, it might be important to insure that sufficient number of patients on various anticoagulants are enrolled in the trial and stratified appropriately so that conclusions regarding the interaction of the platelet inhibitor and the anticoagulants can be drawn. At a minimum, the trial should collect information about concomitant use of the anticoagulants.

7 Surrogate Endpoints

7.1 Definition

Surrogate endpoints are non-clinical endpoints that correlate with clinically meaningful endpoint, or clinical endpoints that are in and of themselves not clinically meaningful but are correlated with ones that are.

Examples of Surrogate Endpoints

- Pharmacokinetic/pharmacodynamic Measures
- In-vivo biomarkers
    - CD4 count
    - Viral Load
    - Glucose Level
    - Cholesterol Level
- Clinical Surrogates
    - Blood Pressure
- Ex-vivo measures
    - MIC (minimal inhibitory concentration) of an anti-bacterial agent
    - ADP-induced platelet aggregation inhibition
- Non-clinical measures
    - FEV1
    - Radiographic findings

For example, hypertension is a surrogate endpoint that correlates with clinical outcome such as stroke, but in and of itself is not clinically meaningful. If a drug could eliminate all the negative outcome associated with hypertension, then hypertension in and of itself wouldn't be a cause for alarm.

Ejection fraction is another surrogate endpoint – in and of itself, it is a non-clinical measure of cardiac function, but is a harbinger of poor outcome if it is compromised.

This is in contrast to non-surrogate endpoints such myocardial infarction, prolonged hospitalization, pneumonia, that are in and of themselves clinically meaningful.

7.2 Need for Surrogate Endpoints

Surrogate endpoints are commonly used in clinical practice to guide treatment decisions. For example, 95% stenosis in a coronary artery may lead to a PCI, high HbA1C might lead to increase in the insulin dose, and active urine sediment might precipitate aggressive immunosuppression in a lupus patient. Because of this, many clinical trials use surrogate endpoints and results of such trials often drive clinical practice.

Example: CAST Study

High rates of PVC's have been known to be predictive of sudden death post myocardial infarction. Several drugs were developed with suppression of PVC's as the goal, with the ultimate goal of reducing death post myocardial infarction. The CAST study was initiated in 1987 with flecainide, moricizine, and encainide, which had been shown to be highly effective at reducing PVC's. At initiation of the trial, there was debate about whether it was ethical to randomize patients to placebo when the drugs had been demonstrated to reduce PVC's. In all, 2309 patients were randomized.

The DSMB stopped the study early because the patients receiving antiarrhythmic therapy had an unacceptably high mortality rate. The RR of death and nonfatal events at 10 months was 4.6 in favor of placebo.

As an aside, the rate of mortality seen in the antiarrhythmic group was lower than historical controls. If it had been deemed unethical to conduct a placebo-controlled trial, then we may still be using these drugs in post-myocardial infarction patients.[2]

However, a surrogate endpoint is never as informative as the clinical endpoint, and in many instances, surrogate endpoint have turned out not to be predictive of clinical response at all. For example, antiarrhythmics that are highly effective at preventing PVC's have been shown to increase mortality. Some antihypertensives do not lower risk of clinical outcome. For this and other reasons, the regulatory authorities (usually) and many clinicians insist on clinical rather than surrogate endpoints.

Surrogate endpoints are highly useful in following situations.

- Phase II, with smaller sample sizes and shorter study durations
- Dose response determination, with multiple arms that may not be large enough to be powered adequately for clinical endpoints
- Disease with slow progression, making the trial is too long for a clinical endpoint (e.g., bone fractures in patients with osteoporosis)
- Diseases with low event rates, necessitating a large trial if a clinical endpoint is used (e.g., stroke in patients with hypertension)
- Subgroup analysis when the subgroup is underpowered for the non-surrogate endpoint

Surrogate endpoint can also be postdictive and used to estimate what the baseline characteristic was pretreatment. This can be useful if adjustments for covariates must be performed.

7.3 Characteristics of a High Quality Surrogate Endpoint

For a surrogate endpoint to be useful, it must fulfill several requirements

- Predictive of outcome
- Sensitive to treatment effect in the same manner as the clinical outcome
- More sensitive or faster than the clinical endpoint

The ideal surrogate endpoint is one that is in the causal pathway.

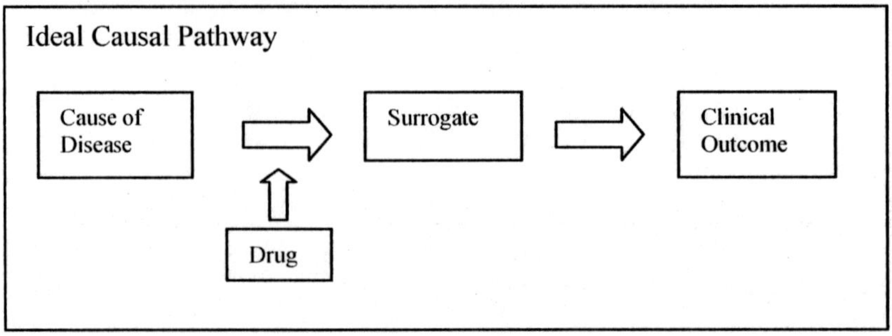

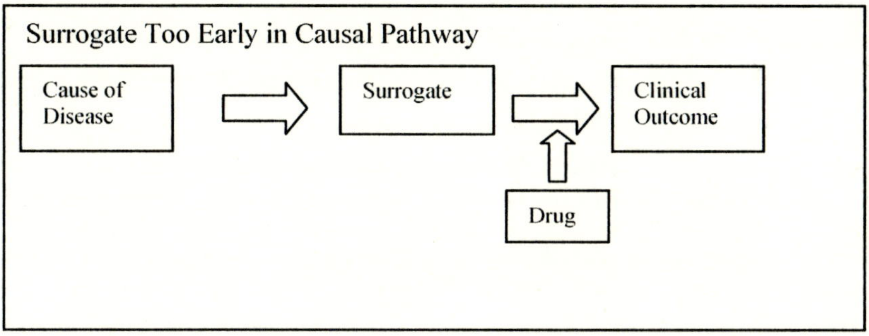

A surrogate endpoint may correlate with disease activity, and may be predictive of outcome without being sensitive to treatment effect. For example, *H. pylori* antibody may be predictive of duodenal ulcers, but antibiotic treatment that eradicates the infection will not reverse antibody positive status.

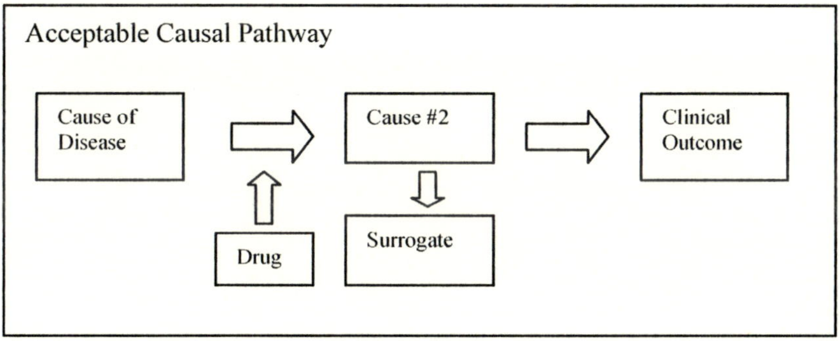

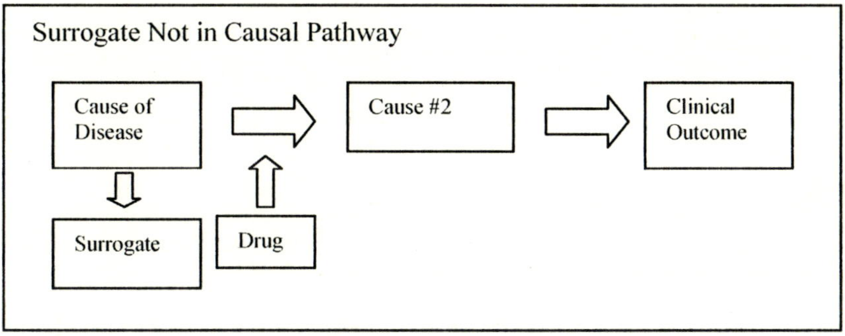

An endpoint may be a good surrogate for one drug but not be a good surrogate for another drug with a different mechanism of action. For example, ejection fraction may be a good surrogate for efficacy in congestive heart failure patients for vasodilators but not for pFox inhibitors. As another example, coronary artery patency is predictive of outcome with thrombolytics, but not when compared across therapeutic classes against thrombolytics plus a IIb/IIIa inhibitor.

Obviously, for a surrogate to be of utility, it must be more convenient (calculated glomerular filtration rate *vs.* measured glomerular filtration rate, or ST segment resolution *vs.* angiographic patency), or faster (bone mineral density *vs.* hip fracture rate), or more sensitive (ejection fraction *vs.* mortality), or precede an irreversible outcome (rejection on biopsy *vs.* organ rejection).

7.4 Validating a Surrogate Endpoint

Validating a surrogate endpoint is difficult, and akin to validating an animal model of a disease. Ideally, it should have been shown to have good positive predictive value (drugs that had an effect on the surrogate had an effect on clinical endpoint); have good negative predictive value (drugs that did not have an effect on the surrogate failed to show clinical effect); be understood in terms of its place in the causal chain relative to the drug. Also, the validation ideally would have been performed with a drug with a mechanism of action similar to the new drug. These conditions are rarely fulfilled, particularly for a drug in a new class, and the selection of a surrogate endpoint is often a difficult judgment call. Even surrogates commonly used in clinical practice such as ejection fraction are often not validated surrogates.

8 Additional Topics

8.1 Individual *vs.* Aggregate Endpoints

The endpoint with the highest sensitivity and specificity for evaluating individual patient may not be the endpoint with the highest sensitivity and specificity for discriminating between active and inactive therapy in a clinical trial.

For example, ACR20 is better than joint count in discriminating clinical response on an individual patient basis. A patient may have 2-3 joints improvement but that in and of itself may not be of clinical significance if the patient is otherwise doing no better. It is partly because joint count alone tends to overestimate response that ACR20 was chosen by ACR.

However, if joint count is responsive to therapy, and is a more sensitive measure of drug activity, it might be a good endpoint for a clinical trial meant to assess whether a drug has activity or to compare doses (e.g., in Phase II trials). In other words, a patient might not consider improvement in joint count in absence of other improvements significant, but it can nonetheless be a useful surrogate endpoint for drug development.

8.2 Clinical Practice *vs.* Clinical Trial Endpoints

A practicing physician uses many signs, symptoms, and laboratory measurement—all of which can be considered to be endpoints—in his practice. However, the endpoints that are well suited for clinical practice may not be the best for clinical trials, and vice-versa.

In terms of selecting an endpoint, the considerations in clinical practice include:

- Ease of use
- Speed of use
- Cost of use
- Ability to discriminate findings to guide therapy
- Ability to discriminate finding to render prognosis
- Rich in descriptive data, even if they can't be well captured quantitatively

The considerations for clinical trials include:

- Ability to standardize across sites, even if it requires training
- Ability to document results
- Ability to reproduce results and methods at different sites, countries, times

So, for example, breath sounds alone, while it may be of high clinical utility in guiding therapy, is difficult to use in clinical trials because it is cumbersome to record (in cases where it is important that it can be audited later, they breath sounds would have to be recorded on a tape recorder), subject to differences in technique, and difficult to quantify.

On the other hand, measure glomerular filtration rate of FACS analysis is much too cumbersome to use on a routine basis but may be an ideal endpoint for trials.

8.3 Objective *vs.* Subjective Endpoints

Objective endpoints are endpoints measured quantitatively or with an instrument, such as walk distance, joint count, or viral load. Subjective endpoints are softer endpoints that require much judgment by the patient or the investigator such as pain, dyspnea scale, and quality of life.

Ironically, even though purely automated quantitative endpoints are often considered unacceptable as endpoints because they are surrogates, subjective endpoints that are difficult to standardize and reproduce are often faulted because they are too reliant on clinical judgment.

The distinction between objective and subjective endpoints are blurry, and well-designed and standardized subjective endpoints are acceptable, although in general, objective endpoints are preferred because they are more amenable to aggregate data collection, analysis, and interpretation.

8.4 Clinical *vs.* Non-Clinical Endpoints

Not a clinical endpoint in itself:	Clinical endpoint:
Infiltrate on chest x-ray Low pO2	Clinical diagnosis of pneumonia, based on both of the following: 1) Clinical judgment of pneumonia *and* 2) Either infiltrate on CXR and/or low pO2

Non-clinical endpoints are often considered to be surrogate endpoints.

In some instances, a non-clinical endpoint can be transformed into a clinical endpoint with the addition of clinical discretion. For example, a chest X-ray by itself may not be a clinical endpoint, but a clinical diagnosis of pneumonia, which must be base don an X-ray among other parameters, can be a clinical endpoint:

8.5 Static *vs.* Dynamic/Change *vs.* Cumulative Change

Static endpoints are endpoints that are absolute, such as ejection fraction or blood pressure. Dynamic endpoints are endpoint that measure change.

ACR20 is an example. It is possible to derive the dynamic endpoint from static endpoint but not the other way around.

Some endpoints measure the disease severity at one timepoint, such as joint pain, while others are cumulative endpoints, such as amount of joint erosion.

8.6 Remission *vs.* Response

Traditionally, response means that a patient has had a good response so that the disease is nearly or completely gone but that the patient remains on the drug, while remission suggests that the disease itself was modified and is doing well even after the drug has been discontinued.

8.7 Need for Intervention as Endpoint

Sometimes need for intervention can be an endpoint, such as need for procedure such as rescue PTCA. This is somewhat controversial, with some researchers arguing that procedures that are shown to be of benefit should not be considered an endpoint.

Need for rescue medications can also be an endpoint. An example would be need for systemic steroids.

In a similar vein, the ability to reduce the dose of a medication with recognized side effects, such as reduction in systemic steroids, can be an important endpoint.

In some indications, the ability to wean patients off another drug may be of significant benefit. For example, systemic steroids have detrimental long-term effects. There can be several approaches to this, such as immediate mandated decrease or mandated lowering of the dose of steroids over time.

Weaning studies must be designed carefully because they can lead to confounding, however, especially if one group has higher number of patients who wean but the number of exacerbations rises. It can then be difficult to tell whether the drug is of clinical benefit, and whether the patients who were deriving the benefit were the ones who were having the exacerbations – it might be acceptable to have 10% increase in eh severity of the disease if those same patients were the ones who could wean from systemic steroids, but unless the study is designed carefully, it may be that the patients who are benefiting are different from the ones who are getting worse.

8.8 Pharmacoeconomic Endpoints

Reduction in resource utilization, such as hospitalization or days of ICU care can be a surrogate for severity of the disease in addition to being a pharmacoeconomic endpoint.

8.9 Disease Endpoint *vs.* Symptom Endpoint

It is important to recognize that an endpoint can be a disease endpoint or a symptom endpoint. For example, most Co-2 inhibitors have a disease indication such as relief of symptom in patients with rheumatoid arthritis, and a symptom indication, for relief of acute pain. Pain endpoints can cut across multiple indications.

8.10 Area Under the Curve

With an endpoint that is continuous, the endpoint can be an area under the curve endpoint. This can increase the power of the study, much as with repeated measures method. Area under the curve is an attractive endpoint intuitively, because the course of the disease over time is an important clinical endpoint in many chronic diseases.

8.11 Quality of Life Endpoints

Quality of Life is considered one of the more subjective endpoints. It is also called patient reported symptoms. It is a valuable endpoint for many diseases, but prone to methodological weaknesses.

8.12 Durability of Response

Especially for a waxing waning disease such as psoriasis, and for chronic disease such as rheumatoid arthritis, durability of effect is an important component of a drug's effectiveness. In many diseases, a treatment that induces a remission is the ideal drug.

Also, it is sometimes desirable to show that a drug continues to work over time or perhaps that it gets better over time. For that, it may be necessary to continue a placebo-controlled period, which can be difficult.

Alternatively it is possible to compare short duration to long duration (like Raptiva- also include in analysis section)

8.13 Drug Sparing as an Endpoint

The goal of some clinical trials is to decrease or obviate use of another drug, typically because the other drug has toxicity. For example, lengthening time to dopamine medication, or other type of rescue as an endpoint can be an endpoint. Essentially, the clinical endpoint is initiation of medication.

This is related to but different from a drug sparing endpoint, such as lowering go dopamine or lowering of steroids–this is complicated because it is sometime difficult to demonstrate that the benefit is being maintained at the same time. It may or may not be the case that the patients who are improving also the same ones decreasing the medication. The average clinical outcome may improve and there might be a reduction in the dosage of the other medication, but these may be occurring in different patients.

It is also difficult to know if the reduction in dose results in reduction in toxicity in a linear fashion. For example, it may be that reducing average dose by 50% has only 10% reduction in safety problems, so reduction of 50% might not mean much.

Of course, if the drug that is being downtitrated has a better safety and/or efficacy ratio, then it is not beneficial to reduce the dose. For example, reducing need for PTCA has been used in several acute coronary syndrome trials, but it is not clear that reducing the need for PTCA is clinically meaningful. So when a dose reduction of another drug is an endpoint, one is implicitly comparing the two drugs, and asserting that one drug is better

8.14 Cure *vs.* Treatment

Some drugs cure the disease–they fundamentally changes the pathophysiological process such that the disease no longer exists. Antibiotics are a classic example of this. Others treat the disease such as the underlying cause of the disease remains but the symptoms and effects of the disease may be reduced or eliminated.

8.15 Symptom *vs.* Disease Modification

Some drugs treat the symptoms, such as pain, others treat the biological effects of the disease, such as long-term progression of joint erosion, and others do both.

8.16 Induction of Remission *vs.* Maintenance

Some drugs induce the remission of a disease when it is actively flaring, others prevent or reduce the recurrence of flares.

8.17 Improvement *vs.* Prevention of Progression

Some drugs improve the disease – such as restoration of vision, while others prevent or slow progression. This is an important distinction. For example, a drug that prevent further damage in stroke might need to be given as early as possible, and a clinical trial may fail unless the patients are treated early, while a drug that enhances regrowth of nerve tissue might be given long after the stroke.

8.18 Speed of Onset of Effect

For certain diseases, such as a very painful disease, onset of action would be much more important than for other disease, such as osteoporosis.

8.19 Durability of Effect

Disease-modifying agents have a long durability of effect, as do drugs with long pharmacodynamic half-life such as alefacept. Others, such as Flolan, have a very short durability of effect, with sometimes devastating consequences.

8.20 Tachyphlaxis

Certain drugs—nitrate is a classic example—lose part or all of their efficacy over time, as the body comes attenuated to it, or the counter-regulatory process kick in.

8.21 Efficacy upon Retreatment

Some drugs only work once they do not work as well on re-administration. Classic examples include biologics such as streptokinase or murine antibodies. For an indication such as acute myocardial infarction, where few patients have more than 1 or 2 episodes, this may be acceptable.

---

[1] Appelbaum FR, et al. Bone Marrow Transplantation or chemotherapy after remission induction for adults with acute nonlymphoblastic leukemia. Ann Int Med 1984, 101:581-588.

[2] CAST Investigators. Preliminary report: effect of encainide and flecainide on mortality in a randomized trial of arrhythmia suppression after myocardial infarction. New England J. of Med 1989; 321:406-12.

Chapter 5: Assignment to Treatment Groups and Randomization

1 Rationale for Control Groups

Broadly speaking, clinical research can be classified into descriptive, associational, and explanatory.

1.1 Descriptive

A single type of clinical phenomena—such as height—measured a single time in a group of people can be described even in the absence of any other data. Indeed it can only be described. For example, the mean, standard deviation, 10th percentile, 90th percentile, can all be described.

A natural history study is an example of a study that is largely descriptive. From such a study, it is possible and common to obtain valuable information, such as rate of death, malignancies, and other clinical events are, along with a confidence intervals. (It should be noted that the confidence interval is not just a function of the disease or the make-up of the population, though. It is dependent on the sample size and the event rate as well.)

However, a natural history study can also describe the correlation between patient characteristics and outcome. These however would be associational findings, not descriptive. It is rare that a study is purely descriptive. Ironically, an uncontrolled safety study (clinical trial) where all patients receive an intervention, and inadequate historical controls exist is an example of a study that is mostly descriptive.

In many instances, an uncontrolled study is the only feasible one and in many instances descriptive studies can yield valuable information.

1.2 Associational

When data on two or more parameters are available, it is possible to describe association or correlation among them. Examples include

- Height *vs.* sex
- Height *vs.* success in basketball
- Height now *vs.* height later
- Height *vs.* sex *vs.* age
- Height *vs.* sex *vs.* age *vs.* success in basketball

Many epidemiological and observational studies fall into this category. Associations can be between intervention and outcome, risk factor and outcome, among risk factors, etc.

1.3 Explanatory

When data on two or more parameters are available, and certain other conditions are met, then it is acceptable to infer a causal relationship among them. The requirements for this are

- Patients are assigned an intervention (as opposed to patients deciding on the intervention for themselves)
- There is a comparator group who were not assigned an intervention
- The intervention occurs earlier in time than the outcome of interest
- There is a difference in outcome between those who received the intervention and those who did not

Examples include:

- Randomized to drug now *vs.* blood pressure later compared to placebo group
- Assigned to surgery now *vs.* survival later compared to adequate historical control group

Some examples of conditions that do not fulfill the requirement for causal association include:

- Blood pressure now *vs.* drug later
- 100% of patients with tumor receiving surgery (no comparator group) *vs.* survival later

There are certain exceptions where the association is so convincing—such as tobacco smoking and lung cancer—that a causal inference is appropriate even if all these criteria are not met, but these are rare.

Pyramid of Inference

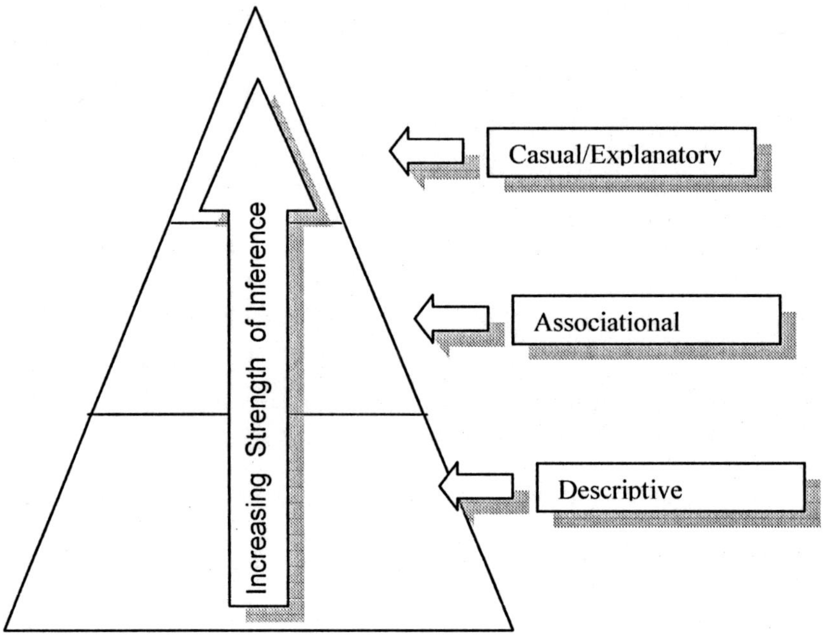

Causal/Explanatory: Generally requires randomized prospective clinical trial, with an intervention (drug, device, surgery, etc.) In certain cases, methods other than randomization may suffice. Pivotal Phase III clinical trials fall into this class.

Associational: Most observational and epidemiological research falls into this class, as do most safety finding in clinical trials. Associational inference posits a correlation between two factors, but does not assert a causal relationship.

Descriptive: This is most common in case series and clinical trials with a single arm and no controls. It describes the findings, using parameters such as mean, median, and standard deviation.

2 Types of Controls

In order to draw associations or explanatory inferences about an intervention, there must usually be two or more groups. Usually, there are two groups: one that receives the intervention and one that dose not. The group that does not is the control group.

Strictly speaking, it is possible to draw associations between clinical parameters even if there is not a formal control group, so long as there is heterogeneity in both parameters. This is accomplished by modeling, and is discussed briefly in a later section.

- Assigned Controls
    - Randomized
        - Simple
        - Blocked
        - Stratified
        - Adaptive (falls into two categories)
            - Dynamically balanced for baseline characteristics
            - Dynamically based on response
    - Alternate assignment
    - Assigned on basis of parameter
        - Entirely on basis of parameter: on intended outcome measure
        - Matched controls
        - Adaptive (falls into two categories)
            - Dynamically balanced for baseline characteristics
            - Dynamically based on response
    - Historical Control
- Unassigned Controls
    - Case controlled
    - Cohort controlled
    - Cross-sectional
- Uncontrolled
    - Heterogeneous intervention or clinical parameter
    - Uniform intervention

For controlled studies, the types of comparators that may make up the controls include the following.

- Placebo control (including on a background therapy)
- Sham control
- Other doses
- Active control
- No treatment control
- Historical control

3 Assigned Controls

3.1 Background

Assigned controls mean that the treatment was determined not by the patient or ht treating physician but the investigator responsible for the overall study. This removes an important source of bias that can threaten internal validity of the study: namely, that there is almost always a reason why certain patients received a therapy or an intervention and why someone didn't. It could be as subtle as the rate of speech in an asthma patient or slight diaphoresis in a myocardial infarction patient. It is almost impossible to adjust for the baseline differences if the treatment is not assigned, because the unmeasured covariates are impossible to fully capture.

Assignment is generally performed by randomization in most clinical trials. However, there are important exceptions to this, as discussed below.

3.2 Randomization

Randomization produces groups that are balanced for both known and unknown risk factors and covariates. Because of the complexity of clinical status and response, it is impossible to match patients exactly on each one of infinite number of variables that might affect the course of disease and likelihood of response. Randomization, if the sample size is adequate, insures that the treatment and control groups are adequately balanced with regard to baseline characteristics.

Most randomization schemes are now generated with a random number generation computer program, and the assignment is usually made via interactive voice response system. It is still possible, however, in small studies, to utilized paper based randomization. In order to minimize the bias that may be introduced if the enrolling physician can guess the order of randomization, it is important to keep the assignment truly random.

The types of randomizations are described below.

3.2.1 Simple

This is straightforward pure randomization. Each patient is assigned to treatment group based on chance alone.

3.2.2 Blocked

Blocked randomization is based on a randomization code that is balanced within each block. So for example, in a 200 patient study, each group of 10 patients may be randomized to 5 placebo and 5 active treatments. This insures that if the study is terminated in the middle, there won't be a major imbalance. It also minimizes the potential of bias that may be introduced if most patients at the beginning of the study receive one type of treatment and vice versa. This is particularly a concern if standard of care is changing rapidly and enrollment is expected to take a long time, or if the disease is affected by seasonal changes.

Blocking also decreases variability slightly, but not enough to make this a major consideration.

Blocking sometimes is also used to mean that patients are matched for baseline characteristics. To avoid confusion, I will refer to this as matched randomization and it is discussed below.

3.2.3 Stratified

Stratified randomization is used when a baseline characteristic is known to have a strong influence on the outcome of interest. For example, patients with anterior myocardial infarctions are known to have worse prognosis than patients with inferior myocardial infarctions.

In a very large trial, most baseline characteristics will be balanced across the treatment groups on their own, but for small or moderate trials, there is a risk that one or more characteristic will be unbalanced. To minimize this risk, randomization is performed separately for the subgroups. The result is that the two groups have equal numbers of patients with the characteristics.

Some of the baseline characteristics that often can affect outcome or endpoint include the following. Clinical judgment and analysis of data from previous studies in the indication is important in deciding the stratification variables.

- Which site the patient was enrolled in
- Severity of baseline disease
- Subtype of disease
- Age
- Concomitant medications

If it is important to prespecify a secondary endpoint for a subgroup, it is also necessary to stratify the groups.

Unfortunately, unless the study is very large (in which case there is less need to stratify), it is possible to stratify on a handful of parameters because the randomization blocks become too small.

3.2.4 Adaptive

Strictly speaking, adaptive randomization is a combination of randomization and parameter based assignment, but we will discuss in this section. Adaptive randomization generates assignment based on a factor that changes during the course of the study.

Dynamically balanced for baseline characteristics
Adaptive randomization can dynamically balance important covariates as the randomization proceeds. As previously noted, stratification on a more than a handful of variables is impossible with most studies. A randomization computer program can keep track of the number of patients with certain covariates that have been randomized to each treatment arm, and change the probability of assignment to the groups based on the patient being randomized.

This type of randomization is extremely useful in insuring that the groups are balanced for important known characteristics, and decreases the overall variability of the study.

Dynamically based on response

In certain types of studies (e.g., dose ranging, device, Bayesian), the randomization can dynamically integrate the response to drug or intervention and change the likelihood of assignment to the groups based on whether the previous patient(s) responded or not. This is generally useful only in situations where the response is rapid – for example, short term pain relief or defibrillation studies—and can be assessed between each randomization.

The advantage of this randomization scheme is that it reduces the sample size, and can maximize the likelihood that the most number of patients receive a beneficial therapy in the course of the trial. In some instances, this type of randomization is the only ethical type of study that should be conducted.

One weakness of this scheme is that it ignores time effect bias: it assumes that patient characteristics, response, and clinical standard of care remain constant over time.

3.3 Alternate assignment

In older clinical trials, assignment was sometime based on a fixed pattern. For example, the first patient would receive A, the second B, the third A, the fourth B, etc. Because it is easy to predict the assignment, there is risk of bias on the part of the enrolling physician or patient. Alternate assignment is rarely used or needed, and even in situations where 100% enrolment of every sequential patient is insured.

3.4 Assigned on basis of parameter

Assignment based on a parameter rather than by randomization is rarely used, except as part of adaptive randomization. In general, randomization is superior in that it can balance for unknown covariates.

In very small studies, or in specific situations with unique ethical or logistic constraints, non-randomized assignment might make sense.

3.4.1 Entirely on basis of parameter: on intended outcome measure

Patients can be assigned to therapy based on their intended outcome measure. For example, patients with severe lupus flare with glomerular filtration rate below 30 can all be assigned to treatment and patients with glomerular filtration rate above 30 can be assigned to control. Regression discontinuity analysis can be used to analyze results of such randomization. It is counterintuitive, but by analyzing whether the regression line for the pre and post treatment values is discontinuous, it is possible to determine whether the drug is effective in the treated group or not. Counterintuitively, this type of analysis is not affected by regression to the mean or effect of the severity of the disease on outcome.

This type of assignment is highly unorthodox and probably has not been used in clinical trials but is invaluable for certain situations. For example, if it would be unethical to perform a placebo controlled study in a certain disease patients because a therapy has become standard of care already, but FDA will not grant approval without a trial, this type of design may be the only possible option. The disadvantage is that this scheme will increase sample size by 2.75-fold.

3.4.2 Matched controls

Sometimes called block design, this is a trial where each subject is matched to a patient who is similar before the randomization is performed. The matching is done on sex, age, and other baseline characteristics thought most likely to affect disease progression and response to drug. For example, patients are permitted only to enroll in pairs, and each pair must have same sex, age, and duration of disease. An extreme example would be studies done on identical twins. The idea is to minimize variability and imbalances between the treatment groups.

Matched randomization is generally not practical, and with advent of computerized adaptive randomization systems, no longer necessary.

3.4.3 Adaptive

This was discussed above.

3.5 Historical Controls

Historical controls may be perfectly acceptable in cases of diseases known to have a certain outcome. For example, they could be used in a disease known to be terminal, or a disease such as ponchocerciasis that never remits on their own.

In general, however, historical controls are treacherous because confounding is almost certain. Some of the confounders include:

- Change in practice pattern over time
- Differences in patient population
- Difference in collection of endpoint

In general, it is almost impossible to replicate the conditions under which the historical data was collected, and historical controls should be avoided.

4 Unassigned Controls

In the absence of assignment, matching can generate control patients. This is typical in epidemiological studies. However, secondary and exploratory analysis in clinical trials will often rely on unassigned controls. For example, nested case control analysis may be used to examine biomarkers.

Interpretation of nonrandomized, nonassigned data is discussed in detail in the analysis section, but the brief descriptions of matched controls are listed below.

4.1 Case controlled

Case controlled studies match patients with and without an outcome of interest. The risk factors are examined in the matched patients. For example, 60 year old men with prostate cancer and X, Y, Z characteristics are matched with 60 year old men without prostate cancer and the same X, Y, Z characteristics. Their risk factors are then examined, for example with data from draft physical examination.

4.2 Cohort controlled

Cohort controlled studies match patient with and without a risk factor. They are then examined for the outcome of interest. For example, women who have high and low fat diets may be matched for other characteristics and followed to examine the outcome of breast cancer.

As an aside, most randomized prospective clinical trials are a subtype of cohort studies.

5 Uncontrolled

True uncontrolled studies (i.e., no historical controls) can be descriptive. In case of uniform intervention – for example very patient receives drug—it is not possible to draw association between the intervention and outcome.

In cases of heterogeneous intervention or risk factor, correlation can be drawn with an outcome because in effect, such studies serve as their own controls. Univariate or multivariate analysis can be performed even in the absence of a clearly identifiable control group so long as the risk factor is heterogeneous. For example, a correlation can be drawn between amount of exercise and coronary artery disease.

6 Other Considerations

6.1 Randomization by Site or by Group

In some instances, where it is logistical difficult to randomize patient by patient, it is possible to randomize by larger units. For example, hospitals can be randomized to new clinical care protocol or the old one on a hospital-by-hospital basis.

6.2 Unequal Ratios

The ideal randomization is usually 1:1, but 1:2 or other randomization ratios can be used if logistic or other reasons require it. With 1:2 or 2:3 randomizations, increase in sample size required in minimal—less than 10%.

Chapter 6: Blinding and Reducing Bias

1 Overview

Apart from randomization and sampling, blinding (also called masking) is the most important determinant to the validity of the study, and one of the most important ways in which bias can be minimized.

In order for a study to draw valid conclusions, it must be free of bias- that is, systematic error that will make one treatment or another superior when in fact there is no difference between the two. The goal of a clinical trial is usually to determine whether difference in a single factor—presence of absence of the intervention or drug—can causally alter the outcome. In other words, all other factors should be identical, including patient population, concomitant treatment, assessment, follow-up, etc.

Any difference in any of the factors between the two groups is bias, and greater the bias, the more difficult it is to attribute any difference in outcome to the intervention alone. Bias can be classified into several categories.

Systematic bias is a systematic error that affects both the control and active arms equally. They include training effect, better health care due to patients being in the study, and time bias. All of these can affect the generalizability of the study, but because they affect both control and treated arms equally, do not usually affect the ability to draw conclusions regarding the differences between the arms (internal validity). In some cases, there can be an interaction – for example, results of a complicated surgical or interventional procedure may only be applicable to tertiary care centers with highly advanced staff—but this is the exception. This topic is discussed in depth in a later section.

Differential bias does represent a threat to internal validity of a study because such biases affect the apparent efficacy of the treatment. One important differential bias is differences in baseline characteristics. These can clearly introduce bias. Randomization, stratification, and in some cases, multivariate adjustment can address the bias from imbalances in baseline characteristics at the beginning of the study.

The other differential bias is difference not at the initiation of the study but during the course of the study, including differences in how the patients are assessed, placebo effect, differences in dropout rates, etc. Some of the differences arise as result of the drug itself – such as differences in efficacy and safety that results in patients being treated differently—but more commonly, it is because knowledge of treatment arm can lead to different treatments.

<table>
<tr><td rowspan="3">Systematic Bias (e.g., training effect)</td><td colspan="3">Differential Bias</td></tr>
<tr><td rowspan="2">Bias at Initiation (e.g., imbalance in demographic factors)</td><td colspan="2">Bias during trial</td></tr>
<tr><td>Bias due to effect of the drug (e.g., greater efficacy not requiring symptomatic medications)</td><td>Bias due to knowledge of treatment assignment (e.g., more exertion on treadmill)</td></tr>
</table>

Without blinding, there are multiple potential biases that can be introduced, but one of the most important is the placebo effect. For many diseases, the response can be affected by the knowledge that the patient is receiving the drug. This is particularly true when the endpoint is subjective, such as symptoms, or dependent on effort, such as the 6-minute walk. Placebo effect is great, and the randomized blinded trials make the implicit assumption that efficacy – as opposed to effectiveness is the goal. In real life, of course, the patients will receive the benefits of placebo effect as well as the pharmacological effect. Placebo effect can exist even in active control trials and dose-ranging trials, since patients who are on high doses or on investigative therapy might believe the drug to be superior. Blinding will not eliminate the placebo effect but will equalize them.

Knowledge of treatment can also affect the patient's willingness to stay in the study and can result in differential dropout effects.

In addition, the knowledge of the treatment assignment can bias the physician assessment, such as ACR20 score or safety events. It can also affect the quality of care the patient receives, or likelihood of receiving concomitant medications.

Blinding is to reduce differential bias – other biases, such as bias from better care, will not be affected by blinding, and neither will the better safety because of closer care given to the patients (c.f. with effectiveness section)

Using sustained response or repeated measures to reduce placebo response rate.

2 Types of Blinding and Dummying

2.1 Types of Blinding

In general, open label refers to the patient knowing which treatment arm he has been assigned to. The terms single blind, double blind, and triple blind are used somewhat inconsistently, but in general, means that one or more of the following groups are blinded: patient, investigator, or sponsor.

In practice, blinding is more nuanced, and the possibilities include the following.

- Blind patient – blinding the patient minimized the placebo effect
- Blind Investigator
  - Blind treating physician– blinding the investigator minimized differences in the way the patients are treated. It also decreases the chance that the patient will be inadvertently unblended
  - Blind the assessing physician – sometimes the treatment cannot be blinded (surgery *vs.* sham surgery) and a blinded assessor is needed
  - Blind site personnel – ideally, all members of the healthcare team at the site will be blinded. In some instances, it is necessary to unblind the pharmacist or another member of the team
- Blind Sponsor
  - Everyone – ideally, everyone at the sponsor would be blinded
  - CRA's
  - Everyone exception safety group for reporting
  - Everyone except monitor

2.2 Special Procedures

Special procedures may be necessary for suppositories, eye drops, skin patches, etc. For example, for patches, the patients may need to wear a covering that prevents them from seeing which patch they are wearing. Drugs with a characteristic color may need to be administered in opaque IV lines. Drugs that have a low pH and sting on injection should be matched with a placebo that has a similar pH and also stings.

Certain drugs have a pharmacodynamic effect that can unblind the drug, such as PTT, lymphocyte count, etc. Ideally, the lab results will not be shown to the investigator, but in cases where it is important to monitor the laboratory value and adjust the treatment accordingly, a separate physician can be assigned to handle the task.

In some cases where the drug has to be prepared at the site, it is sometime necessary to unblind the pharmacist in order to prepare the drug.

2.3 Dummying

When an IV drug is being compared to an oral drug, or where the drugs are very different in appearance and overencapsulation is not possible, it might be necessary to use a double dummy process, where a placebo is prepared for each of the drugs and each patient receives one active and one placebo drug.

3 Unblinding Due to the Drug's Effects

No matter how well the blinding process is designed, if the drug has a characteristic side effect such as an infusion reaction, or marked efficacy, the patients and investigators might be able to guess the assignment. In such cases, bias is inevitable. If this is expected, it is advisable to prospectively collect information regarding whether the patients and the physicians were able to guess the treatment arm.

4 Breaking the Blind

4.1 Breaking Blinds in Emergencies

In some cases, a patient will have an adverse event and in order to insure appropriate care to protect patient safety, the blind must be broken. In these cases, the blind should be broken and the personnel who need to know the information should be informed. The blind break should also be recorded.

4.2 Breaking blind for Regulatory Reporting

Many sponsors will break the blind for serious unexpected adverse events in order to determine whether to report the event to regulatory authorities. This also allows close monitoring of the safety event pattern in the trial.

4.3 Disclosing Assignment to DSMB

For trial s that have a DSMB, the blind will be broken for them usually by an independent third party statistician, in order foe them to assess the safety.

4.4 Breaking the Blind for Administrative Reasons

Although generally not advisable, it is possible to break the blind to trigger an independent event, such as preparation for the next clinical trial. In such a case, extreme care is necessary to preserve the blind.

4.5 Partial Unblinding for Administrative Reasons

In some cases, the blind may be broken after the primary endpoint has been reached, but only a select group of people may be made aware of the results. This might be the case, for example, if 6 month efficacy is the primary endpoint but 12 month efficacy endpoint is an important secondary endpoint. Unblinding at 6 months might allow initiation of the next trial or regulatory filing, but the sites and patients would not be told of the assignment until after the 12 month time period in order to minimize the bias in the study.

Chapter 7: Intended Comparisons and Powering/Sample Size

1 Comparisons and Powering

The most common goal in a trial is to compare the difference between two groups. However, in some cases, the goal may be to compare several groups, and in other cases it may to establish equivalence across two or more groups. In other cases, particularly in safety studies, the purpose may be to describe the characteristics of a particular group of patients rather than to perform a comparison.

In all of these cases, it is important to estimate in advance the appropriate size of the study in order for the study to be scientifically and ethically acceptable. A study that is too small will not answer the scientific question, and will subject the patients to risk without a valid scientific reason. A study that is too large is scientifically bad form, wastes resources that could have been directed toward another scientific question, and also exposes patients to unnecessary risk.

⇨ Truth ⇩ Study Results	Drug does not work (Null Hypothesis is true)	Drug works (Null hypothesis is false)
Study is negative (Accept Null)	1-α (Confidence Level) Probability of True Negative	β (Type II Error) Probability of False Negative
Study is positive (Reject Null)	α (Type I Error) Probability of False Positive	1-β (Power) Probability of True Positive

In designing and powering a study, and in drawing the boundary for accepting or rejecting a hypothesis, the goal is to maximize the power and confidence level while minimizing Type I and Type II errors.

An underpowered study is the worst design flaw possible, since it likely will not lead to the answer that the investigator is looking for, and it is not just unnecessary expenditure of resources but more importantly, potentially exposes patients to risks for no purpose. Furthermore, a study that is underpowered can results in a false negative results, which can often be misinterpreted by the lay physician as proof that the therapy is not efficacious.

The appropriate sample size of the study is dependent on the following factors.

- Comparison
  - The comparator group
  - The type of comparison (equivalence, superiority, etc.)
  - The number of comparisons
  - Equal *vs.* unequal sample sizes
- Statistical Bar
  - Alpha
  - Power
  - Type of tail – one sided or two sided
- Endpoint
  - Distribution of primary variable
  - The expected event rate in the control group
  - Variability in the endpoint
  - Type of Endpoint
- Drug or Therapy
  - The expected effect size/clinically meaningful difference
  - Variability in bioavailability and pharmacokinetic/pharmacodynamic of the drug/patient
- Expected Drop-out Rate

Each will be discussed in this chapter.

2 Types of Comparators

2.1 Comparator Group

The comparator group may be made up of one of several different types, as listed below. Although in and of itself, the comparison group doesn't directly affect power or sample size, it does have enormous impact on variability and other factors that do, so are listed here.

- Placebo control (including on a background therapy)
- Sham control
- No treatment control
- Other doses
- Active control – appropriate dose
- Self control (crossover)
- Historical control (can be any of the above)

2.1.1 Placebo control

Placebo control is one of the most common types of controls. Ideally, the patients in the control group receive drug that is indistinguishable from the active drug in appearance. In practice, this might require dummy pills (see below). In general, placebo control is the most desirable type of control, and allows for the cleanest comparison.

Trials that are conducted on background therapy (for example, all patients in all groups receive methotrexate, and in addition, they receive drug or placebo) are considered to be placebo-controlled trials.

2.1.2 Sham Control

In cases where placebo control is not possible – for example with surgical procedure trials, it may be possible to perform sham controls. For example, if it is not ethically feasible to perform placebo intravitreal injections in a study of an intravitreal drug, it may be feasible to perform procedures that mimic an injection (that to a patient is indistinguishable from an injection) but does not subject the patient to the possibility of endophthalmitis.

2.1.3 No Treatment Control

In cases where even sham control is feasible, no treatment control may be the only option. This would of course mean that the patient is not blinded. Examples would be surgical or device trials.

2.1.4 Other Doses

For dose ranging studies, some of the control groups can be other doses of the drug. In trials with multiple arms, there are special considerations with respect to powering and analysis, discussed below.

2.1.5 Active Control

In some studies, the control arm may be another drug known to be effective for the disease. Of course, the most scientifically rigorous studies would always have a negative control (placebo), active control (a drug known to work), and the test groups. However, in clinical trials, this is rarely feasible from a logistic viewpoint.

In many cases, the drugs will need to be double dummy and/or the drugs may need to be overencapsulated.

Also, if the intention is to use the results of the trial for registration or a comparative claim, the comparator drug will need to be studied at the maximal approved dose. In the case of a drug that is a standard of care but has not been formally approved for an indication, the choice of comparator could be problematic if the goal is registration, since the FDA is generally reluctant to approve drugs on basis of a comparison against an unapproved drug. If the current standard of care drug has been studied in well-controlled adequate trials, it may be possible to convince the FDA that the body of evidence still shows that the drug being tested is better than placebo. In those cases, the burden of proof is on the sponsor, and the endpoint used will need to be similar.

2.1.6 Dose Ranging *vs.* Active Control with Dose Ranging in Both

A study that compares multiple doses of one drug against multiple doses of a comparator drug can be performed in special cases.

2.1.7 Self Control (Crossover)

Crossover can be mixed with one or other controls above, but the comparison is being made against the same group for each dose or treatment.

2.1.8 Historical Control

Historical control is problematic in many cases, but may be the only alternative in some conditions. Every attempt should be made to find a group that is comparable to the one being studied, and appropriate adjustment made for differences in patient characteristics.

2.1.9 Comparator Regimens

In some cases, it will be necessary to compare regimens of drugs against other regimens. For example, different cancer therapy cocktails may be compared against other cocktails. Scientifically, this is perfectly acceptable, and in the past, FDA has accepted these types of designs, but recently, they have expressed some reluctance.

2.2 Ethical Issues

Randomization to placebo, particularly when there is an approved or accepted therapy available, is controversial, and more controversial than is often recognized. This is particularly true outside United States, where placebo is not as well accepted (see Declaration of Helsinki Para 29).

In many countries, and in certain indications, the relevant clinical question is not whether a drug is better than placebo but rather whether a drug is better than the current standard of care. In fact, in many countries, this is the standard that a new therapy must meet before it is granted registration. In contrast, the regulatory and legal bar for new drugs is superiority to placebo in the United States.

In many cases, the question of whether to use placebo is a judgment call. Diseases with irreversible sequelae—such as death or permanent loss of function—is more difficult to perform placebo-controlled trials in. Diseases with highly efficacious therapies are also difficult to perform placebo-controlled studies in.

Excerpt from the Helsinki Declaration

The benefits, risks, burdens and effectiveness of a new method should be tested against those of the best current prophylactic, diagnostic, and therapeutic methods. This does not exclude the use of placebo, or no treatment, in studies where no proven prophylactic, diagnostic or therapeutic method exists. See footnote

The WMA hereby reaffirms its position that extreme care must be taken in making use of a placebo-controlled trial and that in general this methodology should only be used in the absence of existing proven therapy. However, a placebo-controlled trial may be ethically acceptable, even if proven therapy is available, under the following circumstances:

- Where for compelling and scientifically sound methodological reasons its use is necessary to determine the efficacy or safety of a prophylactic, diagnostic or therapeutic method; or

- Where a prophylactic, diagnostic or therapeutic method is being investigated for a minor condition and the patients who receive placebo will not be subject to any additional risk of serious or irreversible harm.

All other provisions of the Declaration of Helsinki must be adhered to, especially the need for appropriate ethical and scientific review.

2.3 Types of Intended Comparisons

The intended comparison can also have an enormous impact on sample size. The possible comparisons include:

- Superiority
- Noninferiority
- Equivalence
- Descriptive

2.3.1 Superiority

Superiority is the most common type of comparison for several reasons. First, most trials are for new therapies that are intended to advance the treatment options for a particular disease. In general, this means being superior in efficacy, or sometimes being superior in safety to the current drugs or treatment options, although not always so (for example, it might improve convenience – instead of a complicated multi-step infusion, 5 sec bolus). Second, superiority studies are generally smaller than the other types of studies.

For a superiority study, the intent is to demonstrate that a drug or therapy is better than a comparator arm. Traditionally, this requires that the p value for the comparison between the two arms be less than 0.05, which is equivalent to saying that the likelihood of the observed difference happening by chance is 1 in 20 or less.

2.3.2 Equivalence

Equivalence studies are meant to demonstrate that a therapy is similar to the comparator arm.

At the first glance, it might seem that this is opposite of the superiority criteria. Intuitively, one might think that $p > 0.05$ might be an appropriate. However, not meeting the high bar for showing a difference doesn't mean that the opposite is necessarily true. For example, $p=0.10$ still makes it much more likely that the two treatment arms are different than that they are alike. It just doesn't meet the high bar that is required to meet the statistical test.

If that were the only issue, then setting the $p > 0.95$ might be the appropriate test for establishing equivalence. However, another major issue is that the incentive to conduct a well-run trial is great when the goal is to show a difference (show a small p value) – the opposite is the case when the goal is to increase the p value. P value goes up with higher variability, which means that a highly insensitive endpoint could fail to show a difference between groups.

Sloppy trials can also result in the results looking similar – for example, sloppy randomization that results in patients mixing up their drugs could make the treatment arms appear similar.

In order to address these issues, the traditional way of establishing equivalence relies on the confidence intervals of the groups being within predetermined limits. Or stated another way, equivalence criteria require that the confidence interval between the arms fall within certain parameters. As an example, one equivalence criterion previously used by the FDA mandated that the new treatment maintain at least 90% of the treatment benefit that the comparator drug conferred.

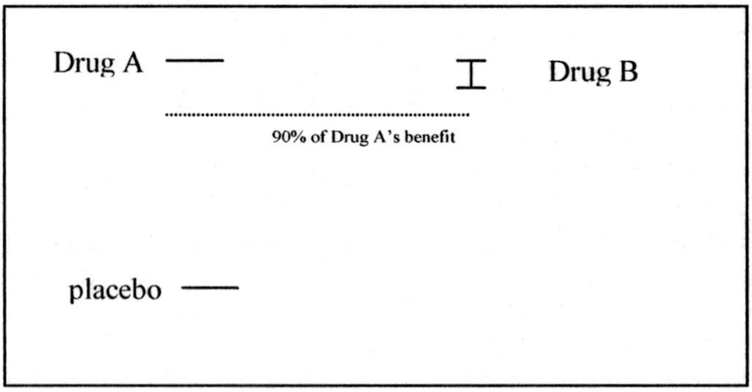

Using a confidence interval overcomes some of the above issues because C.I. becomes smaller as the quality of the study and the sample size increases.

Equivalence criteria are based on both the statistical considerations and clinical considerations. For example, if Drug A has been established to reduce hospitalizations from 30% a year to 5% a year, it might be reasonable to assert that a drug that could reduce hospitalizations to 5% (C.I. 0%-10%) with confidence interval of 0%-10% would be equivalent. If however, Drug A reduces mortality from 30% to 5%, it is not likely that a drug with confidence interval of 0-10% would be accepted as equivalent, since it could potentially double the mortality rate compared to Drug A. More likely, it would have to either demonstrate 5% (C.I. 4%-6%).

Because the confidence intervals need to be very small in general to demonstrate equivalence, equivalence studies as a rule are much larger than superiority studies.

It should be noted that statistically, it is impossible to prove that two groups are identical – it is only possible to show that the difference between or among groups is likely to be less than a certain amount. This is because statistics is based on estimates that are based on a sample (or a subset) of the population. In essence, clinical trials are similar to a survey – it relies on a subset of patients for data, and the conclusions are based on the subset of patients. Just as no poll taken before an election is 100% guaranteed to be exactly the same as the election results, it is not possible to say with 100% certainty that results seen in two groups are the same.

2.3.3 Noninferiority

Equivalence usually requires that the confidence intervals be vanishingly small. Because of this, it is often impractical to set the sample size large enough to show equivalence. A more realistic goal is to show noninferiority. Noninferiority requires that a therapy be not worse than the comparator arm. It is in general a lower bar, as the criteria for the C.I. is often less. For example, FDA will often accept 50% preservation of the comparator drug's benefit as acceptable criteria for non-inferiority.

Also, if the drug is better than the comparator drug but the sample size would be too large to show superiority, then noninferiority may be an acceptable option. For example, if Drug A (the comparator drug) lowered mortality from 30% to 5% (C.I. 0%-10%) and Drug B (the drug being tested) lowered mortality to 2% (C.I. 0%-7%), B would not be statistically superior to A but may meet the noninferiority criteria.

2.3.4 Correlation

Some studies are intended to demonstrate a correlation between factors rather than to test a hypothesis. This is most common in pharmacokinetic/pharmacodynamic studies or mechanism of action studies.

2.3.5 Dose Response

Dose response analysis can be analyzed using a trend analysis. This can establish a relationship between the doses and placebo without direct comparison between an active arm and placebo. It is also more powerful than simple pairwise comparisons.

2.3.6 Descriptive

For single arm studies, particularly for single arm safety studies, the sample size is often calculated on the C.I. that is desired or on the number of patients required to have a reasonable chance of observing rare events.

The sample sizes required to have a reasonable likelihood of seeing at least one event given a true event rate of 1/1,000 and 1/100 are shown in the table below.

N	Probability of observing an event that occurs 1/1,000 patients	Probability of observing an event that occurs in 1/100 patients	95% CI
25	.025	.222	0,0.14
50	.049	.395	0,0.07
100	.095	.634	0,0.04
1000	.632	>.999	0,0.003
10,000	>.999	>.999	0,0.0003

Rule of thumb

If none of the n patients show event of interest, then the upper 95% CI is approximately 3/n

(Louis, 1981)

For detecting safety events, the length of follow-up is often as important as sample size, because many safety events occur as a function of time. Indeed, events such as torsades de pointes that occur during loading of the drug are an exception rather than the rule, and sample size alone cannot guarantee adequate detection of safety events.

Regulatory requirements call for a minimal number of patients in the safety database that varies with the intended use of the drug. For example, the minimal number of patients exposed to a drug intended for chronic use is 1000 for 1 year per intracranial hemorrhage guidelines. This number may be increased if an untoward signal is detected.

2.4 Multiple Comparisons

When there are multiple arms in a study, a global statistical test for differences among the groups followed by individual test for the comparisons between two groups at a time or penalty for multiple comparisons is appropriate. Often, however, these penalties are not taken, which is controversial. For example, two doses of a drug may be compared against a single placebo arm, and the comparisons may be made independently each with an alpha of 0.05 – this is not strictly acceptable. For this reason, it is advisable to only have two groups in Phase III studies.

2.5 Ratio of Randomization

In general, 1:1 randomization is optimal. However, there are cases where it might be desirable from logistic or ethical considerations to use a different ration. For example, it may be necessary to collect safety data from treated patients, or it may be desirable to examine subgroups in the treated patients, or it may be desirable to have a more precise estimate of various measurements in the treated group.

1:2 or 2:3 randomization doe not result in significant loss of power.

3 Statistical Bar: Power, Alpha, Sided, and Randomization Ratio

3.1 Background

The statistical bar that is set, which in part reflects the degree of risk or confidence the investigator is willing to assume, has an important role in sample size.

3.2 Alpha

The alpha is the amount of false positive rate one is willing to tolerate. Traditionally, this has been set at 0.05. This is arbitrary, but for most purposes, is appropriate.

3.3 Power

Most pivotal studies are powered at 0.8 or 0.9. Power is the likelihood of detecting a difference if it truly exists. At 0.8 (or 80% power), one is likely to see a difference if a true different exists in 80% of the cases. Of course, this means that the likelihood of a false negative is 20%. Power is a judgment call, often driven by practicalities of a feasible sample size.

Traditionally, powering is based on the estimated true effect. For example, if true effect of a drug on MS is to reduce the incidence of an MS flare by 20%, then the in order to insure 80% power, the study must reach $p<0.05$ even if the observed reduction is less than 20%. This is because if the true rate is 20%, then half the time the observed reduction will be greater than 20%, and half the time it will be less. If the study were powered so that it reached statistical significance only if the observed reduction was 20% or greater, then it would fail to reach statistical significance at least half the time.

There are cases, however, where if the observed benefit does not reach a certain value, then the drug is of little clinical benefit. For example, if another MS drug reduces the incidence of MS flares by 25%, then a drug that statistically significantly reduces flares but with an observed point estimate of 10% may not be of clinical utility.

Additional consideration is the size of the database necessary to detect rare or infrequent safety events.

Also, if it is important to assess efficacy or safety in one or more subgroups, or if one or more of the secondary endpoints is very important, the sample size may need to be adjusted upwards to insure that sufficient data is available.

The rate of dropouts and missing data, along with imputation methods, can have a profound effect on sample size.

Also, the sample size depends on underlying event rate, magnitude of the benefit, variability, and the placebo rate. Placebo rate can be affected greatly, especially if there is a subjective component of the endpoint, by unblinding (such as stinging on injection), the randomization ratio (2:1 *vs.* 1:1), the intensity of follow-up and improved care (such as better wound care in a wound healing trial), and the provisions for rollover trials – if there is great incentive to be a responder so that the patient can roll over into the follow-on trial.

Positive predictive value and negative value often determine the size of the studies when there is met medical need. In those cases, whether or not statistical bar is met is not so important as whether the drug is likely to be better than the current available therapies. In other words, if there is a drug for rheumatoid arthritis that induces ACR20 response of 60%, then only a drug that is at least as good as or better than that may be worthwhile. One can perform a comparative study, but more often, clinical judgement calls for the point estimate to appear somewhat equivalent even if the trial is not a true head to head. For example, powering for 90% power with assumption that the true rate is 60% is probably unwise, since that would mean that even 50% ACR20 response might be statistically significant. However, the drug may not be worthwhile in that case. Powering the study to yield a certain confidence interval may be more useful. Or if the decision for go no go is – even if the drug has 50% response, there is 30% chance that its true value is 60% or greater, so we will go ahead with Phase III, or if the safety offsets the efficacy, then it may be worth pursuing.

3.4 Type of Tail

One-sided tail indicates that one is only interested if the difference between the two groups is in a certain direction. Two-sided tail indicates that one is interested in a difference no matter which direction the difference is in. In effect, a two-sided test doubles the alpha compared to a one tailed test. For example, a study with a two side test with alpha of 0.05 on each tail is equivalent in size as a study with a one sided tail with an alpha of 0.1.

In theory, if one were only interested in whether a drug is better than placebo, it would be appropriate to perform a one-tailed test. In practice, this is rarely done.

4 Endpoint

Endpoint is extensively discussed in a separate section. The relevant points about endpoints as it related to power is that higher variability increases the sample size, that a non-normal distribution of the endpoint can increase the sample size required (although once the sample size reaches 20 or so, non-normal distribution ceases to matter as much), and that the expected event rate has a profound impact on power.

The expected event rate is often difficult to calculate, particularly because historic data is unreliable – small changes in the inclusion and exclusion criteria can profoundly influence the event rate. It is advisable to be conservative with the event rate assumptions, and to perform sensitivity analysis around the event rate assumptions. For instance, if the sample size would double if the assumed baseline event rate changes by 5%, then the sample size should be increased, or the sample size adjusted in the course of the trial.

A particularly important caveat applies to estimate of the baseline rate that is calculated from historical data. In general, placebo effect should be expected in all studies, and can be particularly pronounced if there is any subjective component to the endpoint. Also, patient sin clinical trials tend to get better care than the average patients, and this can lower the event rate as well.

Rule of Thumb

Sample size can be estimated roughly by the following rule of thumb.

Sample size = 16 x (standard deviation)^2 divided by (difference to be detected)^2

Lehr R, Sixteen s-squared over d-squared, Stat in Med 11:1099-1102, 1992.

5 Therapy

Perhaps one of the most important determinants of sample size is the expected effect of the drug or therapy. Greater the expected effect, smaller the sample size. Study sample sizes are often based on the estimated effect of the drug, which can be based on preclinical data or on an earlier study. If the expected effect size is based on an earlier study, regression to the mean should be carefully considered and the sample size adjusted accordingly. Phase II studies often show a greater effect than Phase III studies because in general, only positive Phase II studies lead to Phase III studies, and therefore there is an inherent bias toward overestimation of the effect size if only Phase II data is considered.

Alternatively, rather than basing the sample size on the expected effect size, the sample size can be based on the minimally clinically relevant difference. That is to say, if it is known for example that a drug would have to show at least a 10% reduction in asthma exacerbations in order to be considered to be of clinical utility, the study sample size can be based on that.

An important note is that when a study is powered for a certain effect, with a certain power, even a lesser difference can be statistically different. For example, if a study has 90% power to show a difference if the true difference is 10% reduction in exacerbations, it must have enough patients to reach p value of less than 0.05 even if the reduction is less than 10%. Obviously, if the true value is 10% reduction, then half the time the actual observed reduction will be below 10% and half above. For the study to have 90% power, it must be able to reach p value of 0.05 or less even in some of the cases when the actual observed value is less than the true value.

If clinical practice patterns will not be changed by a 7% difference with p value of 0.05, then it is not necessary or advisable to power the study to show a statistical difference with that point estimate.

6 Dropouts

A well-powered and designed study should anticipate a certain proportion of the patients dropping out of the study or becoming lost to follow-up. It should be large enough so that even after imputing for the patients who drop out, the study will have adequate power.

Chapter 8: Periods

1 Background

Time and timing plays a critical role in clinical trials.

First, it is the fact that the intervention occurs before the outcome is measured that gives clinical trials the ability to ascribe causality to the intervention.

Second, because practice patterns, outside influences such as seasons, and patient populations can change over time, time can be a major confounder in clinical trials. Because of this, parallel group trials are preferred over non-parallel trials.

Third, because in some cases outcome can be measured during the trial before all patients have been assigned to treatment, and because in all cases clinical development program alternates intervention and outcome measures, timing of intervention and measurement of outcome can greatly impact the scientific rigor and parsimony of the trial.

The types of trial designs with different periods include the following

- Parallel Designs
- Within-patient Designs
    - Crossover
    - Latin Square
- Factorial Designs
- Sequential Designs
    - Individual sequential
    - Drop the loser
    - Play the winner
- Other Periods
    - Run-in
    - Withdrawal

2 Parallel Group Designs

The most typical clinical study design is a simple parallel group design. Patients are randomized into two or more groups, and each group receives different treatments contemporaneously. This is more straightforward way of performing the trials, and usually has the least risk for bias.

The main drawbacks are that the variability tends to be the greatest with parallel design, necessitating the greatest sample size, and that randomization is not guaranteed to eliminate all imbalances in the groups, particularly when sample sizes are not large and/or disease is very heterogeneous.

3 Within-Patient Designs

There are several within-patient designs. In these types of trials, patients are used for more than one treatment type. This has the advantage of reducing variability and therefore sample size. These designs can also be useful when availability of patients is an issue.

3.2 Crossover Trial

The crossover trial is the most common of the within-patient designs. In the simplest crossover design—the two period crossover design–the patients are given one treatment first then another treatment. Multiple crossover designs, where a patient crosses back and forth between regimens are possible but rarely used.

Crossover designs make sense in the following instances.

- The variability between patients is expected to be greater than the variability within the same patient at different times
- Cost is prohibitive for a parallel trial
- There aren't enough patients available for a parallel trial
- The duration of treatment is short

A -> B
B -> A

In general, crossover trials are prone to multiple potential biases, and make some key assumptions that may or may not be true.

First, a fundamental assumption behind crossover trials is that the disease doesn't change over time – in a progressive disease such as MS, this may not be true. However, for a disease with a slow progression or no progression such as allergic rhinitis, it might make sense.

Second, there is an assumption of no carryover effect. The half-life of the drug must be short, and the effect must not have a permanent and durable effect on the disease or disease progression. At least 3 to 5 half-lives are generally required between the periods. Otherwise, the first period and the second period may exhibit major differences. The drug must also act relatively quickly – certainly before the crossover.

If there is a carryover effect, then only the first period may be considered to be valid.

Third, there is an assumption of no time effect. For seasonal rhinitis, the different season might play an important factor in the severity of symptoms.

In addition, there must not be a rebound effect. Also, dropouts are much more problematic in a crossover design than in a parallel group design. Of course, the endpoint of interest must not be permanent – for example, mortality can't be an endpoint because once a patient dies, he can't enter the next period.

Unfortunately, the sample size required to determine whether there is a significant carryover effect is almost always larger than he sample size needed to meet the primary endpoint. (In fact, it is usually the size needed for a parallel group study.)

Crossover studies are often used in pharmacokinetic studies of small molecules in healthy volunteers.

3.3 Latin Square

Latin square designs are similar to crossover study design but with more than two treatment groups. In practice, they are rarely used in clinical trials because the complexity and the potential for carryover effects.

A -> B -> C
B -> C -> A
C - > A -> B

This is an example of a Latin Square design. Latin squares have each treatment represented once in each row and column. This is an example of circular permutation, in that the order of the treatments is always the same A->B->C.

In general, a circular permutation is more likely to introduce a systematic bias, since if one treatment is always followed by another treatment, and there is a carryover effect, it will always occur in the same group.

For a study with even number of treatments, the order can easily be modified to insure that each treatment is followed by each other treatment. This allows an estimation of carryover effect.

```
A -> B -> C -> D
B -> C -> D -> A
C - > D -> A -> B
D -> A -> B -> C
```

```
A -> B -> C -> D
B -> D -> A -> C
C - > A -> D -> B
D -> C -> B -> A
```

For studies with odd number of groups, several alternative exist to avoid the drawbacks of circular permutation: two or more complementary sequences need to be used (preferred), or alternatively an extra group may be added, or extra period may be added (in which case it is not a true Latin square any more, since in a true Latin square each group occurs only once in each row or column).

```
A -> B -> C
B -> C -> A
A - > C -> B
C -> B -> A
```

C -> B -> A B -> A -> C A - > C -> B
A -> B -> C B -> C -> A C - > A -> B

And

A -> B -> C -> B B -> C -> A -> C C - >A -> B -> A

If desired, a treatment may be repeated to see if there is an effect of two sequential treatment periods on the clinical effect.

A -> B -> C -> C B -> C -> A -> A C - >A -> B -> B

Greco-Latin Square is a factorial design within a Latin Square. It is also very rarely used in clinical trials. In that instance, two set of factors are being determines. All the caveats of Latin Square design and the caveats of factorial design apply. An example would be the following.

A – placebo
B – 1 mg/kg of drug
C – 5 mg/kg of drug

1 – traditional counseling
2 – psychotherapy
3 – no counseling

A1 -> B2 -> C3 B3 -> C1 -> A2 C2 - > A3 -> B1

If the full Latin square design is not feasible because multiple periods are not practical, incomplete block design may be used. Conversely, if the availability of the patients is an issue (for example with orphan indications), intensive design may be used.

A -> B -> C -> A -> C -> B
B -> C -> A -> C -> B -> A

A -> B
B -> C
C -> D
A -> C
A -> D
B -> D
B -> A
Etc.

3.5 Dose Escalation

A common within-patient design that is often not recognized as such is dose escalation study design where the same subject receives multiple escalating doses of a drug, where the primary comparison is between doses. This is not uncommon, but the caveats of within-patient designs apply.

4 Factorial Designs

Factorial design involves testing of two different interventions on the same group. A pure factorial design would be two completely unrelated indications being tested in the same patient group – for example, a glaucoma drug in the eye and a dermatitis drug in the hand, in patients who have both diseases.

More often, two drugs are tested for the same or similar indications. For example, the HOPE trial examined the effect of ramipril and of Vitamin E on cardiac events. The Phase IIb Rituxan trial examines different steroid doses and Rituxan doses on rheumatoid arthritis.

Example: Simple 2 by 2 Factorial Design

Group 1 Placebo/placebo	**Group 2** placebo/glaucoma drug
Group 3 Dermatitis drug/placebo	**Group 4** dermatitis drug/glaucoma drug

Factorial designs reduce sample size significantly, and represent an elegant way to address more than one question in one study. In general, the sample size decrease by a factor of 2 for a two factors (2 by 2, or 3 by 3, 4 by 4, etc.) and factor of 3 for three factors (2 by 2 by 2, 3 by 3 by 3, etc.), etc. It is also the appropriate design if one is interested in seeing whether there is an interaction between drugs.

3 by 3 Rituxan RA Phase IIb design

A1	B2	C3
B3	C1	A2
C2	A3	B1

A – no steroid
B – low dose steroid
C – high dose steroid
1 – no Rituxan
2 – 1g Rituxan
3 – 2g Rituxan

The key drawback to factorial design is the potential for interaction, unless interaction is one of the questions being addressed.

Interaction refers to synergy or dis-synergy between two drugs or treatments. For example, cyclosporine plus azathioprin may be more than additive (2 + 2 =5). Alternatively, erbitux and other chemotherapy agents may be less effective than erbitux alone (2 + 2 = 1).

If one is trying to answer the question regarding the efficacy of a combination of drugs relative to each drug alone, factorial design is appropriate. Also, if the objective is to define a dose response surface (similar to dose response curve but with multiple drugs), a factorial design is appropriate, even if interactions exist.

If one is using factorial design to answer two independent questions, interaction can significantly diminish the power of the study. Without interaction, if there are 50 patients in each group, there would be 150 patients per arm to answer each question.

Impact on Sample Size, 3 by 3 Factorial Design: sample size is reduced 2-fold

A1	B2	C3	50	50	50	=	150
B3	C1	A2	50	50	50	=	150
C2	A3	B1	50	50	50	=	150
			150	150	150		

With 50 patient per group,

A *vs.* B *vs.* C compares 150 pts *vs.* 150 pts *vs.* 150 pts

and

1 *vs.* 2 *vs.* 3 compares 150 pts *vs.* 150 pts *vs.* 150 pts

3 by 3 by 3 Factorial Design

```
A1X  B2X  C3X
B3Y  C1Y  A2Y
C2Z  A3Z  B1Z
```

A – placebo drug 1
B – low dose drug 1
C – high dose drug 2

1 – placebo drug 2
2 – low dose drug 2
3 – high dose drug 2

X – placebo drug 3
Y – low dose drug 3
Z – high dose drug 3

Sample size is reduced 3-fold.

With interaction, the n in each comparator group drops down to 50 per group.

As with Latin Square designs, incomplete factorial designs can be performed, although the results are not as powerful.

In the past, logistics were a significant issue with the factorial design. Arranging complex randomization schemes and operationalizing it with paper and envelope system was difficult, and assembling and tracking numerous types of drug kits was unwieldy. However, with modern computerized systems, the logistic complexity is no longer a major issue.

It should be noted that small sample sizes that factorial design allows can magnify issues inherent in any study with small sample sizes, such as imbalance in groups and potential for bias. Some of these are ameliorated by combining the groups for the purposes of analysis, but not all.

2 by 2 by 2 Factorial Design

```
A1X  B2X  B1X  A2X
B2Y  A1Y  A2Y  B1Y
```

A – placebo drug 1
B – drug 1

1 – placebo drug 2
2 – drug 2

X – placebo drug 3
Y –drug 3

Reduction in sample size is 3-fold.

5 Sequential Designs

5.1 Individual Sequential Design

With an individual sequential design study, the results of the control and the active group are analyzed after each patient or periodically after a small number of patients, and the study is modified real-time based on the results.

For example, several different candidate drugs may be compared, and for each instance of a patient responding to a particular drug, the probability of the next patient being randomized to that drug may be increased. This way, maximal number of patients can be exposed to the drug most likely to benefit, and the sample size can be substantially reduced. This can all be done without breaking the blind.

Typically, this type of study is Bayesian in design, and requires an intervention that affects clinical outcome rapidly. For example, such as study may be possible in an acute analgesic study where the outcome can be determined after an hour, but not for an MS study where the outcome isn't known for a year or more, since the outcome influences the randomization scheme.

Although Phase I pharmacokinetic studies might appear sequential in nature, the comparisons in the studies are primarily across dose groups, not against controls, so they are actually non-concurrent parallel group or within-group crossover/modified Latin square trials (if the same patient is dosed repeated with different doses of the drug).

5.2 Group Sequential Design: Drop the Loser

In some studies, it is appropriate to perform an interim analysis in the course of the study and drop one or more of the arms. This can be the result of a DSMB recommendation, or can be planned. For example, if it's not possible to select a single dose based on Phase II data, then more than one dose may be taken into Phase III, and all but one dose group dropped after a certain length of follow-up.

5.3 Group Sequential Design: Play the Winner

The opposite is the play the winner strategy, where additional patients are enrolled into the arm that appears the most promising. For example, a dose escalation Phase I study might proceed with 4 patients per group until some activity of the drug is detected, and additional 10 patients might be enrolled into one or more of the promising arms. This allows more data to be collected in the targeted dose, so that better estimate of efficacy and safety can be made.

6 Other periods

6.1 Run-In Periods

In addition to the comparison periods, where the groups are receiving different treatments, there are non-comparator periods that served other functions.

For example, in some instances, it is useful to conduct a run-in phase. A run-in phase usually is a period before randomization where the patients undergo titration off another medication or gets started on the study drug.

- Drug is not well tolerated by everyone. For example, if the drug causes nausea, it might be useful to conduct a run-in phase, drop out the patients who tend to have the nausea, and then randomize. The side effect would have to be restricted to a small group – it would not make sense to do this unless a subgroup of patients was more susceptible to the side effect, because if the side effect occurred at a fixed frequency in everyone, the incidence would not be lowered. Statistically, this is helpful if even a low dropout would have significant impact on the endpoint

- Patients need to wash out of their current therapy and not everyone will wash out successfully. In this case, the patients would be randomized after the washout. For example, rheumatoid arthritis patients who are taking systemic drugs or psoriasis patients who are taking systemic drugs. One potential issue is that their disease might flare in the washout period. Careful consideration need to be given to whether the patients will be allowed to randomized if they met the inclusion criteria at the beginning of the washout but not at the end.

- Standardization of medication. In some cases, it may be necessary to standardize the medication. For example, if asthma patients are all taking different brands of inhaled corticosteroids, and the protocol calls for steady reduction in their steroid dose, it may be necessary to have a run-ion period to switch the patients to the same type of corticosteroid.

- Establish a baseline. For example, for MS patients, MRI may need to be performed over 6 months of run-in period in order to establish a baseline. This is particularly true for disease in which the endpoint has high patient-to-patient variability but good intrapatient reproducibility. It may be impossible to conduct a reasonably sized study without establishing a baseline. Another example is establishing baseline frequency of events during a specified period such as number of anginal episodes.

- Qualify the patient. In cases where it is imperative to establish the severity of the disease, rather than relying on history. An example is atrial fibrillation, where sometime s the patients report arrhythmia but the arrhythmia symptoms may be caused by anxiety or non-arrhythmic causes. During the run-in period, the patient may be required demonstrate that they indeed have the clinical events.

Similar to a run-in period is an induction period. For example, an atrial fibrillation drug that is designed to maintain sinus rhythm rather than to cardiovert may require that all patients be cardioverted into normal sinus rhythm at the beginning of a study. Similarly, a drug designed to keep patients in remission in lupus may require that patients be induced with another regimen before the study is initiated. Alternatively, a run-in phase may be necessary to make sure that a patient has a certain severity of disease—for example, at least 2 exacerbations of asthma within 6 months, or to standardize or stabilize background therapy or medications.

As an aside, in general, the randomization should occur after the run-in, because to do otherwise would introduce significant bias into the study – if the randomization occurs before the run-in then part of the effect of the arms may be due to the dropouts during the run-in period. Apart from confounding the ability to detect effect of the drug, this also significantly lowers the power to detect differences between the treatment arms.

6.2 Open Label Follow-up Period

After a study has concluded, patients can often be rolled over into an open-label follow-up study. This is helpful in collecting additional long term safety data. In addition, patients with chronic disease who are responding to therapy may be best served by continuing the therapy.

7 Length of Follow-Up

The length of follow-up is complicated decision. Most drugs exert a maximal effect after a length of treatment. Also, if the drug is to prevent progression, such as multiple sclerosis, a certain length of time may be required to show a difference. Also, the clinical significance may be in doubt if the benefit is shown only for a short length of time for a long term disease – such as 3 month relief in symptoms for rheumatoid arthritis.

The other significant factor in the length of follow-up is the dropout rate. In some cases, longer follow-up results in decreased effect size because of dropouts. The etidronate study in osteoporosis suffered from this. It showed an effect at one year but the effect was lost, at 2 years, partly as result of dropouts.

Chapter 9: Patient Selection, Site Selection, and Sampling

1 Disease as an Intellectual Construct

Diseases are intellectual constructs. Although there are real differences between bronchitis and pneumonia, between psoriatic arthritis and rheumatoid arthritis, between classic macular degeneration and occult macular degeneration, all diseases lie on a spectrum, and the decision where to draw the line between one "disease" and another is a judgment call.

This is an important point, because one common mistake in clinical development is to pursue treatments for "diseases" without recognizing that disease classifications change over time and the appropriate population of patient for study should only be partially defined by the current classifications of disease. Rather, the decision on which patients to enroll in a study, particularly for completely novel classes of therapies should be guided primarily by pathophysiology and data on the particular treatment being tested. For example, sepsis might represent a heterogeneous group of biological phenomena, and a reason for so many drugs failing in sepsis trials may be failure to appropriately classify the subgroups of patients. Alternatively, hypertension, diabetes, and coronary artery disease have long been considered separate diseases, but given the unified view of metabolic syndrome that is now emerging, an anti-inflammatory drug that affects metabolic syndrome in general may positively affect all of these diseases.

Categorization of diseases are based on a number of criteria, including:

- Physical or histological manifestations
- Concurrent symptoms or other diseases
- Prognosis and natural history
- Response to treatment

For example, a disease that mainly affected the kidney, such as glomerular nephritis would usually be classified in a different category than a disease that manifest mostly in the skin. However, if many patients experienced a constellation of symptoms that often went together, such as with lupus, the disease may be classified as one.

The most common way to classify disease is by response to therapy. In fact, diseases that may be very different in pathophysiology and clinical manifestations may be classified as the same disease if the treatment is the same—or more commonly, if there are no good treatments for any of them. An example would be schizophrenia, a disease with manifestations that range from catatonic to paranoid schizophrenia. These diseases are classified together partly because they respond to similar therapy.

This is because physicians often take the pragmatic approach and prefer to classify diseases based on their treatment options. For myocardial infarctions, it way not necessary to distinguish as rigorously between ST elevation myocardial infarction and on-ST elevation myocardial infarction before thrombolytics were shown to be effective in one and not in the other. Now, what was previously one disease is considered to be two, or at least two variants.

It is therefore important to think carefully about the "disease" that one is targeting with a clinical trial. It may require expanding the trial beyond the normal confines of a disease – such as lumping CABG, PTCA, and stroke patient together—or limiting the trial to a subgroup of patients such as classic or occult AMD.

In choosing a patient population, the "indication" can be lumped in different ways. For example, it can be lumped by symptoms – everyone having joint pain, for example. Or it can be lumped by having enough of a constellation of potential symptoms that are often seen together – such as lupus. Or it can be lumped by pathophysiological criteria, such as a positive blood culture for an organism.

Alternatively, it can be lumped by causation. For example, patients with tuberculosis may have pulmonary or gastrointestinal manifestations. However, causation is often fraught with challenges because although it is common to assign a single cause to diseases, there is never just one cause – every disease is the result of interaction of environment, genes, and other factors. For example, though *H. pylori* is considered to be the cause of ulcers, many people are infected with the organism. Patients are more susceptible to H. pylori infection if they have Type O blood type, so ulcers are result of complex interaction between multiple factors. Similarly, Whipples's disease is thought to be caused by *T. whippelli*, but many people harbor the organism. The disease is caused by the interaction of the organism with the immune system in susceptible individuals.

Phenylketonuria is considered genetic disease, but if the natural levels of phenylalanine were extremely low in most of our diet, and most people were homozygous for the recessive PKU gene, then the disease may be considered to be result of abnormal diet. If 99% of the population had a mutant versions of CCR5 that kept HIV in chronic dormant state, and there were multiple viruses in the HIV family that was ubiquitous in the population, then AIDS might be considered to be caused by a mutation rather and HIV virus.

So for the purposes of defining diseases for clinical trials, causes of the disease should usually be thought of a risk factor rather than a cause. And defining a disease by response to treatment or by manifestation often makes more sense than defining it by causes or risk factors unless the trial is intended to be a prophylactic trials. This avoids the questions such as "does someone who has an infection without manifesting it have the disease?"

2 Sampling is a Major Limitation of Clinical Trials

In most randomized trials and studies outside clinical research—such as agricultural trials or consumer research studies—random and unbiased sampling is a critical aspect of trial design and conduct. A great deal of thought and effort is expended in an attempt to obtain a truly random, or at least a representative sample, of the population being studied.

A nonrepresentative sample does not reflect the overall patient population, and can limit the generalizability of the study results. Unfortunately, in clinical trials, random sampling is usually impossible. A significant bias is unavoidable when patients are recruited into clinical trials. At a minimum, clinical trials exclude patients who are unable to give informed consent, but also tend to exclude the sickest patients, the most noncompliant patients, etc. There are often biases in that patients from different socioeconomic classes may be more or less likely to enroll – for example, those who can't afford the medication or treatment on their own might be more likely to enroll, or patients who can't afford a phone may be excluded from a trial that requires a phone follow-up.

A nonrepresentative sample in and of itself is an issue but more importantly, it can affect the results of the study or the risk benefit analysis. Patients in a biased sample may have a different natural history of disease – for example they may have a more severe course than the population at large, which would tend to overinflate the magnitude of benefit of the drug. They might also have a different efficacy or safety response to the drug. These can have significant consequences for the overall risk benefit of the drug.

The patient population is almost never truly representative of the patient population at large, and is probably the greatest weakness of randomized prospective clinical trials.

3 Heterogeneity of the Population

3.1 Variability and Validity Trade-Off

Selecting a patient population that is homogeneous usually reduces variability and therefore the sample size. This is because different subpopulations may have different natural histories and different responses to the drug—for both efficacy and safety. Selecting a homogeneous patient sample for a trial is often important in reducing the size of the study and increasing the likelihood of a positive trial.

However, one of the most common methods for decreasing heterogeneity is to limit enrollment to a subset of the patients with a disease or a condition, also limiting the generalizability of the study's results. For example, if patients with only lupus nephritis were enrolled in a trial, then the probability of showing a benefit may be significantly higher than if all lupus patients were enrolled, because the patient population is less heterogeneous and therefore the variability is lower. However, whether the drug would work in non-nephritis patients would not be addressed.

In addition, recruiting a select group of patients can increase logistic difficulties in finding and recruiting such patients in the trial.

3.2 Confirm Diagnosis

Another important way of decreasing heterogeneity is to institute strict criteria for confirming or establishing diagnosis. For example, retinal angiogram might be sent to a core laboratory to confirm the diagnosis of classic AMD. Or documentation of prior chemotherapy might be required to insure that the patient has refractory cancer. Or a run-in period might be used to confirm that the patient does have at least on exacerbation of asthma in a 6 month period, to confirm the severity of the disease.

3.3 Run-in period

Run-in period can be used to decrease heterogeneity in many ways. It can be used to confirm severity of the disease as was mentioned, to confirm that the patient can tolerate the medication, or to standardize background therapy. For example, patients receiving several different types of beta-blockers might be moved to one consistent beta-blocker before the study is initiated. A run-in period might also be used to insure that the disease is in a stable phase or that the background therapy doses are constant before stating the study. Alternatively, a run-in period might be necessary to insure a consistent stage of disease – for example, patients in chronic atrial fibrillation might be cardioverted during the run-in period.

If a run-in period is used, it is generally advisable to make sure that the randomization occurs after the run-in period, to avoid confounding.

3.4 Pharmacogenomics and Biomarkers

For well-understood diseases, it might be advisable to segregate the patients on the basis of biomarkers or pharmacogenomic markers. This is not completely different conceptually from segregating on the basis of clinical or other parameters. With new tools available to assess gene expression, protein levels, integrin expression, etc. the options for subtyping patients has become far wider.

4 Selecting Patients to Include

4.1 Background

One of the most important considerations, and one that take tremendous clinical and scientific judgment, is choosing the population that is likely to benefit from the therapy being tested. In order for a patient to benefit from the drug, he must have the disease being targeted, must have reversible disease or be at risk of having progression, must have the disease as the result of the pathophysiological path that the drug affects, and must not be at high risk of adverse events from the drug. Often, these criteria are not satisfied. The patient may be misdiagnosed with the disease, may have disease that is burnt out, may suffer more harm from the drug than good, etc.

The length of the disease, the stage of the disease (flaring or quiescent), degree of homogeneity in the population, background therapy, concomitant medications, etc. are all critical considerations.

4.2 Relationship to drug's mechanism of action

The mechanism of action postulated for the drug should be aligned with the patients who have the disease. For example, if the drug works by inhibiting T-cells, it probably would not be advisable to test a B-cell modulating agent in the disease. Of course, the caveat is that the pathophysiology of disease is always incomplete, and that the mechanism of the disease may be different from what is expected. Rituxan and rheumatoid arthritis is a case in point. However, it is in general advisable to follow the science and pathophysiology.

4.3 Likelihood of Having an Event

Importantly, in order for a trial to show a difference between the treatment groups, there must be either an improvement in the treated group, or les of a decline in the treated group. In the latter case, the untreated group must be at high enough risk of experiencing a clinical event, or else the trial will not be able to show difference. For Phase II studies, patient populations are often enriched in order to reduce the sample size.

For example, for a moderate size rheumatoid arthritis trial with an endpoint of joint erosion, it would be important to enroll patients who show at one erosive joint because otherwise the patients are unlikely to experience sufficient number of erosions to make the trial adequately powered.

4.4 Likelihood of Responding to Therapy

The patients must have reversible disease or at risk of getting worse in order for the intervention to have an effect on outcome. The amount of tissue or organ at risk must be sufficient so that there is something left to save. Alternatively, the tissue insult must be reversible such that the drug can restore function.

For example, the length of disease is important, because it is often easier to treat diseases at early stages than at the end. Also, some diseases cause irreversible damage to organs, such as macular degeneration with scarring of the retina, and irreversible loss of myocardium in myocardial infarctions.

Diseases at advanced stages are also often multifactorial, and it may be difficult to treat these patients. For example, some of the sepsis trials might have failed because they targeted patients who were too sick and in multi-organ failure, such that intervention that might affect the original cause of the disease was unable to save the patient.

4.5 Patients with Greatest Unmet Need

An important consideration is the unmet medical need. In general, of course, development of a drug or therapy for a disease without adequate current therapy is more desirable than one for a disease or a therapy with effective drugs or therapies.

4.6 Recruitability and Feasibility

An important consideration when deciding on the patient population is the recruitability. The inclusion exclusion criteria can have a significant effect on the number of patients eligible for the trial. For example, excluding patients on NSAIDs for an AMD trial can make the trial extremely difficult to recruit, since NSAID use is common among the elderly.

Although homogeneity in the patient populating is a desirable goal, this must be balanced against practical considerations of recruitability.

In addition, the patient must be logistically be able to participate in the study: he must be able to give true informed consent, he must be able to come in for scheduled visits, he must be able to perform the necessary procedures. Unfortunately, the feasibility requirement can often introduce a bias in studies: indigent patient without transportation or telephone may be unable to participate in the study.

4.6 Diagnosability

The population selected must be clearly identifiable by reproducible selection criteria. Ideally, they would be objective, such as a laboratory test, but clinical diagnosis based on objective standards is acceptable.

4.7 Matching Population with Endpoint

Also, the choice of patient population and the choice of endpoint are intimately linked, and one must be chosen with consideration of the other. A common situation arises when a disease has a waxing and waning course. If the endpoint is induction of remission, then the patients should be defined to include patient who are having a flare, who are likely to eventually resolve their flare with treatment, and who are less likely to resolve the flare without treatment. An example would be patients who are having an acute flare of ulcerative colitis. (It is important to keep in mind that these patients will experience regression to the mean, as is discussed below.)

Similarly, if the endpoint is a prophylactic endpoint, such as for vaccines or broad-spectrum antibiotics intended for empiric and emergent treatment, then the population will not be a set of patients who have a disease but are at risk of acquiring a diseases or experiencing a negative outcome (such as septic shock). Examples include patient s with high LDL levels or patients who are having quiescent lupus. The major challenge in such trials, which tend to be very large, is that it is important to have a good understanding of the risk factors.

5 Patients to Exclude

5.1 Patients at High Risk and Protected Patients

In choosing the exclusion criteria, the patients at high risk and protected groups should often be excluded.

In particular, the mechanism of the drug might dictate that patients at high risk of a particular type of adverse event should be excluded. For example, patients at high fall risk may need to be excluded from trials of anticoagulants, and patients with positive PPD might need to be excluded from trials of immunosuppressive agents. Also, patients who might not have a higher risk of bleeding or infection but would have catastrophic consequences if they were to have an episode may need to be excluded. An example would be someone who has severe congestive heart failure and in whom a major bleed might lead to hypotension and hypoxia very rapidly.

In the past, elderly patients and female patients (particularly those of childbearing age) were often excluded from trials as a matter of course. Part of this was due to paternalism, and in general, they should not be excluded unless there is good scientific rationale. Minorities have also tended to be underrepresented in clinical trials, and if difference in response or safety profile is expected, it is important to make effort to enroll adequate numbers of minority patients.

Children are often excluded from clinical trials for several reasons. Many drugs have a potential effect on development, consent is more difficult to obtain in children, many diseases are not common in children, etc. In general, it is acceptable to exclude children from clinical trials, unless the drug is expected to be used in children.

Pregnant patients are often excluded as well.

There are certain categories of protected patients, such as prisoners and patients unable to give consent. The inclusion of such patients should depend on the specifics of the study.

5.2 Patients with confounding diseases, conditions, or medications

Many patients have concomitant diseases, and are using different medications. Often, in a clinical trial, such patients are excluded. In general, a careful balance must be struck between including patients who will confound the results and generalizability.

For example, in a mortality trial of cancer patients, it might be advisable to exclude patients with terminal cardiac disease. However, for breast cancer trials, it may be necessary to include patient who have received anthracyclin and Herceptin and have congestive heart failure if such a patient population is a significant proportion of the target population.

Similarly, use of multiple concomitant medications can make clinical trial results difficult to interpret. It may be necessary to prohibit concomitant medications during the course of the trial if it ethically acceptable. Alternatively it may be advisable to study such patients in a separate safety study if the safety data from multiple medications is important, or insist on standardizing the dose and type of medication. At a minimum, the patients should remain on stable doses of medications that might have an effect on the study endpoints.

5.2 Patients with biases

In some cases, it is necessary to exclude patient who would introduce a bias. A common example would be patients who have failed other therapies. In indications where there is an attractive standard of care, it is sometimes necessary to exclude patients who have failed standard of care if the study is designed to test first line treatment. For example, patients who have failed tumor necrosis factor inhibitors may be the predominant group who enroll in a rheumatoid arthritis study even if the study is designed to test the therapy as first line treatment, if it does not exclude patients who have failed tumor necrosis factor inhibitors. These types of exclusion criteria must be considered carefully because on the other hand, if it does exclude them, then the trial might enroll patients who are not eligible for tumor necrosis factor inhibitors, such as patients with congestive heart failure, also leading to a bias.

Many patients have concomitant diseases, and are using different medications. If they have a concomitant condition or are on a medication that can impact the clinical outcome being measured in the study, or impact safety, or ability to follow protocol, the patients should be excluded.

6 Phase II Studies

Often, the ideal patient population in Phase I or II studies are different from the desired Phase III population. The population in Phase III should mirror the ultimate target population closely, in order to maximize generalizability. In Phase II, however, it is often advisable to select a subgroup of patients who are more homogeneous and more likely to have an event.

Because Phase II studies are generally smaller than Phase III studies, it is often impossible to adequately power the study without using an alternate endpoint and/or patient population. (See above chapters for discussion of surrogate endpoints). For example, in acute coronary syndrome, one might select troponin positive patients for Phase II since they are at the highest risk of having an additional coronary event. In an asthma trial, one might select patients with the highest number of exacerbations in the previous year. This type of patient population enrichment can lead to smaller Phase II studies.

An important caveat is that the patient population in Phase II must have similar response to the intervention as the ultimate target population. For example, if troponin positive ACS patients had a disease that was fundamentally different in pathophysiology such that they response to GP IIb/IIIa inhibitors while the patients who were troponin negative did not, then Phase II can be very misleading.

A caveat regarding extrapolation of Phase II results to Phase III is that there will always be subgroups who respond better than others to therapy, purely by chance. Unless this subgroup has been prespecified, it is most likely a spurious result. In addition, as the treatment paradigms change, the patient populations that enroll in later trials may be somewhat different from patients who enroll in earlier trials. Also, a positive Phase II trial in itself can change the willingness of patients to enroll in a trial, so that the characteristics of patients in Phase III study may be different solely due to the Phase II results.

7 Patients Who are Refractory to Other Therapy

In some cases, it is unethical to conduct a placebo-controlled trial because the standard therapy is clearly effective and/or the consequences of the disease are devastating. In such cases, the new drug is often developed as an add-on therapy on top of current standard of care. However, for some drugs, it is not reasonable to add onto the current therapy. The toxicity of the combined regimen may be intolerable, or the drugs may negate each other's effects. An example would be a cancer drug that prevents proliferation of tumor cells and one that depends on proliferation for its effects. Or it is anticipated that the new drug would not be as effective as the current regimen.

In such situations, it is sometimes necessary to conduct the study in patients who are refractory to current therapy. There are several advantages to that strategy. These are likely the patients with the greatest unmet medical need, the lowest regulatory bar.

The major issue is that the patients may be too sick to reap much benefit from the drug. For example, patients with longstanding disease might have lost most function already, and stand to benefit little. Or cancers that have been resistant to all standard therapies may be the least likely to respond to the new drug.

8 Geography and Multicenter Studies

Multicenter advantages include speed, generalizability, and replication, while the inconsistency, increased variability and statistical interaction are disadvantages.

In general, modern clinical trials are multi-center, and often international, simply because recruiting enough patients in a reasonable amount of time requires multiple centers. Having multiple centers decreases the likelihood of having a spurious result due to a systematic bias at one center, or due to practice pattern peculiar to one institution or region. For example, the use of IV nitroglycerin in acute myocardial infarction or use of coumadin post myocardial infarction varies considerably from region to region. Having multiple sites across the country reduces the likelihood that the results would depend on presence or absence of a concomitant medication or a particular practice pattern.

It is not just possible but likely that there will be inconsistencies in a multicenter clinical trial. Practice patterns and patient populations do vary across regions and countries. It is not uncommon, for example, for European or Japanese patients to experience different degree of response to a drug compared to U.S. patients. In addition, purely from chance, it is to be expected that some sites will not just fail to show efficacy but actually demonstrate the opposite effect of the drug compared to the overall study. The probability of at least one center having treatment reversal, alpha of 5%, power 80% is shown below.

Number of Centers	1	2	3	4	5	6	7	8
	.003	.05	.15	.29	.43	.56	.67	.75

9 Biases

There are certain biases that are known. Typically patients who enroll in studies tend to be more motivated and be younger. Patients from academic centers tend to be more severe, complicated patients.

Also, patient characteristic change over the course of the study, particularly in a study with a long enrollment period. Patient characteristic can change as result of good results being announced in another trial. This can affect willingness of the patients to enroll in the study, which can vary by the type of the disease. Over time, the most appropriate patients may be more difficult to find, if they have all already been enrolled. Also, there can be changes between screening and baseline.

Also, it is also important to remember that no matter how tight the inclusion and exclusion criteria, no criteria are tight enough to completely prevent population drift.

However, it is important to avoid regression to the mean. For waxing and waning disease, if patients with the worst current disease flares are selected, it should be anticipated that some patients will improve purely due to natural course of the disease and regression to the mean.

Chapter 10: Dosing and Intervention

1 Background

1.1 Drugs *vs.* Other Interventions

All clinical trials involve an intervention. There are many different types of interventions in medicine, but the most frequent type seen in clinical trials is administration of a drug. Less frequent interventions include devices such as angioplasty stents; surgical interventions such as lung reduction surgery; and therapies such as psychotherapy or biofeedback.

The scope of this book, particularly of this chapter, is mostly limited to drugs. However, many of the principles outlined in the book are applicable to other types of interventions. The focus of this chapter is dosing, and dosing is usually a consideration only with drugs, and issues discussed in this chapter such as half-life and compliance are often inapplicable to other interventions.

Of course, non-drug interventions have other types of issues such as surgical (and other) technique, operator expertise, and standardization that are typically not encountered with drugs. In order for results of clinical trials to be generalizable, the intervention must be reproducible so that the practicing clinician can treat patients in a similar way to obtain similar outcome as in the trial. With non-drug interventions such as surgery, standardization is an important aspect of clinical trial design, requiring similar techniques as the ones used to standardize operator-dependent measurements (discussed in an earlier chapter).

It should be noted that while drugs are usually consistent from batch to batch, and usually contain the same amount of active ingredient, standardization of content and potency is not always a trivial issue with drugs. Standardization can often be an issue for biologics and especially for biologics derived or purified from non-recombinant sources. The latter can have significant differences in subspecies, glycosylation patterns, N-terminal modifications, etc. that can affect pharmacokinetic, pharmacodynamic, clinical efficacy, or clinical safety

In some rare instances, dosing methods such as infusion rate or remaining upright for a certain length of time after dosing (such as for bisphosphates) might require attention to standardization techniques even for small molecule drugs. However, in general, the vast majority of standardization for drugs (such as potency, stability, etc.) is performed during manufacturing process, not during administration.

A key characteristic of drugs is dosing. Drugs can be administered in almost infinite gradations of quantity – from microgram quantities to gram quantities or more. This is in contrast, for example, to interventions such as coronary bypass surgery. There is no such procedure as 2¼-vessel bypass surgery.

Also, there is a continuous relationship among doses for a given drug. For example, 5 mg of a drug generally has more physiological effect than 2 mg of the drug, and 2 mg generally has more physiological effect than 1 mg, and so on. There are exceptions, with some drugs exhibiting a U-shaped response curve, but even in those cases, doses that are close to one another have more similar physiological effects than ones that do not. This continuous relationship has an important consequence: it is normally legitimate to treat doses as a continuous variable, and to perform mathematical manipulations and modeling based on doses.

With some interventions, such as hemodialysis, it is possible to adjust the intervention in a similar fashion. The length of dialysis and flow rate for example, can be varied. In many cases, though, a non-drug intervention has no dose or dose equivalent. Cardiac transplantation, for example, is an all-or-non intervention.

Because of the above characteristic, a study with 3 different doses of a drug is fundamentally different from, and offers more than, a study with 3 different interventions. For example, a study with 0 mg, 1mg, 5 mg, and 10 mg of a statin for the prevention of myocardial infarction's is fundamentally different from a study comparing placebo, statin, cholystyramine, and niacin for the same indication. In the first, the dose groups are interdependent, and the result from one dose group has an impact on the interpretation of the other dose groups. Dose ranging studies define a response curve, and each dose group generates a data point that must be interpreted in context of the other data points. Also, even if there is not a statistically significant difference between any one dose and placebo, the results can still be statistically significant if ANOVA or trend analysis is significant. More importantly, the results from the doses provide information about the untested doses—the doses in between the tested doses. In the second, each arm is independent, and the result of one has little impact on the other and certainly does not allow for interpolation between the groups.

1.2 Objectives

Unlike patient selection and endpoint selection, "dose selection" is a term that can often be misinterpreted. This is because "dose selection" has a colloquial meaning: in clinical practice, a physician often selects the dose of a drug for his or her patients, and "dose selection" refers to the decision-making process of selecting a dose.

In clinical trial design, "dose selection" means selection of a dose or doses to test in a clinical trial for a group of patients, not for a single patient. It includes considerations such as whether to adjust for the differences in weight or other characteristics, dosing frequency to test, whether to titrate the dose to a pharmacokinetic or clinical endpoint, and so on. The dose selected for Phase II or Phase III clinical trial may or may not be same as the dose that an individual clinician decides to use for individual patient in clinical practice. In fact, with pediatric patients, the doses adopted in clinical practice are often those never tested in clinical trials.

Of course, depending on the disease, the endpoint measured, and the quantity of information gathered during the clinical trials the clinician may end up using only the tested dose. This is because the quantity of information available to him may leaves him or her with only a binary choice, that of using or not using the drug.

Unquestionably, a drug that is safe and effective is the goal of any clinical development program, and an appropriate dose that allows this goal to be reached is the hallmark of a successful dosing strategy. However, that is not the sole or primary aim of dose selection and exploration. The primary objectives of dose selection and exploration is to define the efficacy, safety, and convenience curves for a drug in relation to dosing, to define parameters that can affect those curves, and to determine whether there is a dosing regimen or set of dosing regimens that strike the appropriate balance between efficacy and safety. Done well, these can lead to safe and effective dose(s), and importantly, to adequate dose characterization.

Dose characterization refers to elucidation of other pertinent relationships of the doses to clinical or other effects. This includes, for example, characterization of the safety margin, drug interaction, dose-response relationship within a population and subpopulations, dose-response relationship within individual patients, variability in pharmacokinetic among different patients, interaction with food, etc. It also includes determination of the optimal starting dose, individual dose response, and maximal dose for drugs that need to be titrated rather than given as a flat dose.

This is because even if a dose or several doses with a favorable risk benefit profile is identified, a physician in clinical practice will require additional data to utilize the drug. Selection of an appropriate dose in clinical practice requires data and clinical judgment about the trade-off between efficacy, toxicity, convenience, patient population, the degree of unmet medical need, alternative available therapies, and extrapolations about the unknown characteristics of the drug.

So, in sum, successful dose selection and exploration yields information about the relationship between doses and outcome, which in turn can lead to a dose or doses that can be useful in clinical practice.

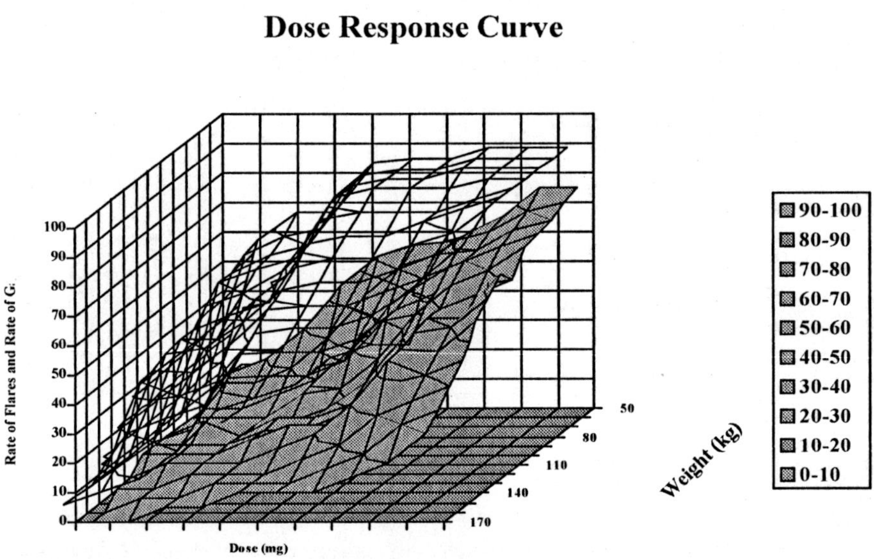

The efficacy and safety curves graphed against weight and dose. The objective is to determine the areas where the curves separate sufficiently to make the drug viable for clinical use.

Of course, collecting and characterizing additional information about a drug and dosing requires time and resources. It is often a temptation to continue to collect additional data, but in many situations, particularly for severe unmet medical need, the dose response curves are defined scantily in order to bring the drug to the patient as quickly as possible. This chapter is concerned with how best to design the trials to test dosing regimens, interpretation of the resultant data, and perhaps most importantly, deciding how much data is enough, and when additional data is necessary.

1.3 Challenges in Dose Selection

The two challenges in dose selection are optimization of the risk:benefit ratio and heterogeneity management. The two are related. Absolutely critical to balancing risk and benefit is assessment of heterogeneity and balancing heterogeneity against convenience and the therapeutic index. Patients' response to a drug, both for efficacy and safety, are heterogeneous. Some patients will respond better, faster, and more completely than others. Some patients will experience more, worse, or more frequent side effects than others.

Patients have heterogeneity, including their underlying disease heterogeneity, metabolism, size, exercise, exposure to sunlight, compliance, sex, age, concomitant medications, race, etc.

In general, more heterogeneous the response, more difficult it is to find the acceptable balance of safety and efficacy. Heterogeneity is important because it is not the mean risk:benefit that is the most important consideration but rather the patients at 10th and 90th percentile. In other words, an effective response in one patient and no effect in another patient is not really equivalent to moderate response in two patients. One noxious event in one patient and no events in 9 others are not equivalent to 10 patients having one mild event each. The power of clinical trials is the ability to generate aggregate data, but the downside is that ultimately the therapy must be administered to a person. For dose selection, particularly when the therapeutic index is narrow, aggregate data must ultimately be dissected into finer data.

The distribution of efficacy and toxicity in the population, as well as whether the patients experiencing the adverse events are the ones exhibiting response, whether it is possible to identify patients in advance who will have the toxicity, whether it is possible to detect events early and to titrate against it, etc. are extremely important judgment calls that must be made in the course of dose selection.

Heterogeneous response can often be made more homogeneous in several ways. The most common method is by customizing dose, often at the expense of convenience. An example is dosing that is adjusted by weight. Alternatively, the dose can be titrated to a clinical endpoint such as blood pressure. Another is to restrict the use of the drug to a subpopulation, or to use different doses in different populations.

There are other important issues in dose selection, such as being able to predict responders and adverse events early. However, balancing risk *vs.* benefit, as well as balancing convenience *vs.* heterogeneity are the critical aspects of dose selection.

Designing the appropriate dosing regimen requires close collaboration among the pharmacokineticist, toxicologist, and the preclinical scientist. In particular, the dosing interval and the initial doses in the early studies must be based on animal data, modeling, and pharmacokinetic data. In the later stages, the dose selection is ultimately dependent on the clinical efficacy and safety profile, but close collaboration with the other functions will lead to appropriate dose regimens being evaluated.

In order to optimize the therapeutic window in the context of heterogeneity and convenience, there are several degrees of freedom or parameters that can be adjusted. They are summarized below.

1.4 Performance Criteria and Constraints on Dose Selection and Exploration

In the simplest sense, the optimal dosing is one that maximizes safety and efficacy. However, it is not possible to find one dose that is effective and safe for everyone. There is no drug without toxicity, and there is no dose without toxicity. The probability of toxicity at the dose may be low, but it is not possible to eliminate the risk completely. The choice must be based on a balance between the two competing factors. And depending on the individual patient characteristics, different doses might strike the appropriate balance for different patients, which is why dose characterization is important.

Of course, convenience and practicability of the dosing regimen are also extremely important facets of dose regimen selection. These are implicit in every dosing strategy, but are often underappreciated. Convenience is more a nice-to-have; it is a necessity that constrains every drug and dosing regimen. If convenience and practicability were unimportant, then drugs could be weight-adjusted, given as a continuous IV infusion, with frequent pharmacokinetic and pharmacodynamic monitoring, for the lifetime of the patient. Such a regimen would maximize the therapeutic index. Convenience and feasibility of the dosing regimen place stringent restrictions on the available palette of dosing regimens.

The performance criteria for dose selection and exploration are that it produces dose relationship curves that are detailed (many data points), wide (explores a large range of parameters such as age, renal function, etc.), and defines a space where there is good separation between safety and efficacy (even while accounting for individual variation) while maximizing convenience.

Of course, the easiest way to define the safety and efficacy curves would be test a large number of doses simultaneously with clinical endpoints. For example, a new statin could in theory be tested using 20 doses from 1 mcg to 5 g, with several thousand patients in each arm with 5 year cumulative myocardial infarction rate and adverse event profile as the endpoint. With parallel dosing, the biases associated with non-simultaneous treatment periods would not be an issue, and with numerous dose arms and ample sample sizes, the dose response curve for safety and efficacy would be relatively easy to define.

This type of dose selection is not possible for several reasons. First, such a design would almost certainly expose large number of patients to a toxic dose. The first step in dose selection is therefore almost always careful dose escalation, with the aim of establishing a range of reasonably safe doses while minimizing risk to subjects. Second, such large studies are generally not feasible logistically and economically. Therefore, earlier and medium stage studies exploring doses are often conducted with surrogate endpoints and/or enriched patient populations that will allow for an estimate of the dose response curve with smaller sample sizes and shorter timeframe.

Third, many drugs do not have a wide enough therapeutic margin and/or have too much variability from patient to patient that a flat dose will not result in a drug with an acceptable safety/efficacy profile. In such cases, dosing that takes into account weight, type of disease, pharmacokinetic, or other factors may be necessary. For this and other reasons, an iterative approach to dose selection is often required. In an early study, it may discovered for example that patients who are heavier respond poorly to the drug, or that patient with low baseline platelet count tend to experience thrombocytopenia with the drug. Later studies can incorporate such information to tailor the dosing regimens, or in some cases, to tailor the studies themselves. For example, if dose response curves are such that an acceptable therapeutic window cannot be defined, pharmacodynamic parameters *vs.* response studies might be necessary. Heparin is an example where a pharmacodynamic parameter (partial thrombin time) is used to define the dosing.

Because of these constraints, dose exploration and dose selection usually proceeds in three stages: initial establishment of safety window, dose exploration (sometimes iterative), and final dose testing/hypothesis-testing. These are consistent with the classic Phase II, II, and III divisions in drug development, and indeed dosing is a major driver for those divisions.

1.5 Components of Dose Selection and Exploration

Dose selection and exploration define the relationship between dose and response. This chapter explores each component of dose response in turn: dose, relationship, and response. Dose includes amount of drug given and ways to quantify the amount, length of administration, titration of the dose, adjustment of dose, etc. Relationship includes a discussion of the latency between dosing and response, standard model, etc. Response includes variability between patients, surrogates, etc.

The specifics of how to investigate various regimens, and how to design clinical trials to gather information about dosing regimens are presented in the next section. In this section, I discuss the considerations that go into selecting the appropriate dosing regimen—route of administration, titration, duration, etc. —and balancing the competing factors that go into that decision.

2 Dosing and Dose Selection

2.1 Quantity of Drug and Adjusting the Dose/Therapeutic Index

2.2.1 Background

In order for results of a clinical trial to be useful to the practicing clinician, it must investigate a defined, reproducible quantity of drug in a fashion that can be replicated by a clinician in practice. The most common way of quantifying the amount is drug by a flat dose, such as 10 mg or 100 mg. A flat dose such as this—same dose for all patients—is the simplest and usually the most convenient. A flat dose is acceptable for drugs that have a wide therapeutic window, where it could be administered without regard to individual patient variations.

However, a flat dose is often unacceptable, most commonly because the therapeutic window is too narrow. For many drugs, there is not one flat dose that will result in efficacy for enough patients while providing tolerable safety. Individualizing the dose almost always results in improved therapeutic index. In some cases, adjusting the dose, such as with adjusting antihypertensive dose to blood pressure, can be accomplished easily enough to warrant non-flat dose. In other cases, a loading dose might be required to provide an onset of action that is rapid enough, such as with antibiotics.

In the post-hoc analysis, relationship of response to other dose parameters such as concentration can often be helpful. For example, in some cases the efficacy may not be evident unless concentration-response, pharmacokinetics-response, or some other relationship is examined. Also, some adverse events may be related more closely to maximal concentration or other parameters than dose.

However, there are multiple other ways of quantifying the amount, including by patient weight, by AUC, by target concentration, and by pharmacodynamic response. Each of these parameters can be related to the response, so that dose-response, concentration-response, and pharmacodynamic-response curves can all be defined.

Broadly, however, the various ways of customizing the dose can be divided into two types. The first is by adjusting the dose for based on baseline characteristics such as weight or P_{450} status. The second is by titrating the dose by response to the drug, such as pharmacokinetic parameters, pharmacodynamic parameters, or clinical response.

Often, clinical trials will test dosing regimens rather than doses against each other. However, for the sake of brevity, "doses" rather than "dosing regimens" will be used in this chapter.

2.2.4 Dose Based on a Baseline Characteristic

2.2.4.1 Physiology Based Dose

Some of the most important causes of variability in drug response are weight, sex, age, and other physiological parameters. Adjusting dose based on these parameters is a relatively easy and practical way of widening the therapeutic window. Weight is a particularly common parameter used for dose adjustment. Weight-based dosing can be based on several different methods of quantifying the patient weight, such total weight, lean weight, or estimated weight.

Similarly, other physiological parameters such as body surface area can be used to adjust the dose. The choice of the physiological parameter depends on the characteristics of the drug, the patients, and the efficacy and toxicity parameters. For example, the drug's distribution profile, such as whether it distributes into fat, can affect the decision on whether to use total weight or lean weight.

With each of the parameters, the dosing can be adjusted on a pure continuous basis, such as mg/kg or by tiered basis, such as 10 mg for patients under 70 kg, 15 mg for patients >70 kg but <100 kg and 20 mg for patients 100 kg and above. Tenecteplase is an example of a drug that is dose-adjusted in this fashion.

2.2.4.2 Adjustment for Metabolism and Distribution

The second most common way of adjusting dose is by metabolism. Genetic polymorphism, especially in hepatic metabolism such as P_{450} metabolism, can have a profound effect on pharmacokinetics, as can acetylation polymorphism in the N-acetyl-transferase. If a drug is known to be excreted renally, adjusting for renal clearance may improve therapeutic window. Less commonly, doses can be adjusted for impaired liver function if it is cleared hepatically.

Similarly, though less commonly, dose might need to be adjusted for factors that affect metabolism, such as serum albumin levels for highly protein-bound drugs.

2.2.4.3 Other Characteristics

Depending on the disease and the drug, other parameters, such as severity of the disease or subtype of the disease can be used to adjust the dose. The risk:benefit ratio might be different for different patients with different severity of diseases, or the subtype of disease might require a different dose to respond physiologically.

In addition, adjustment for diet can be important—for example, diet rich in green vegetables for someone on coumadin. More commonly, though, the diet is adjusted rather than the dose of the drug.

Finally, adjustment for drug-drug interactions may be necessary, as discussed below.

2.2.5 Titrated/Adaptive Dosing

2.2.5.1 Pharmacokinetics-Based Dose

In cases where the pharmacokinetic of the drug is not well predicted solely by weight and physiological parameters, and where the therapeutic window is narrow, it is sometimes necessary to measure levels of drug in plasma or serum and adjust the drug by the pharmacokinetic response. Digoxin is administered in this fashion. Depending on the characteristics of the drug, trough levels, peak levels, or both may be appropriate measures to guide the dose. Also, some drugs might not reach steady state for a prolonged period of time, and multiple measurements of drug levels and multiple frequent adjustments may be necessary when the drug is initiated.

In order to establish a true concentration-response relationship, dosing to a particular concentration rather than correlating resultant concentration to effect is necessary. In other words, a prospective study that examines titrating to the target concentration is necessary to definitely establish the effectiveness of dosing to a concentration. This is more rigorous than a using a post hoc analysis to demonstrate a concentration-response in a standard dose ranging study. The latter is prone to confounding, because even if the patients who achieved highest concentration exhibited the best response, confounding factors cannot be ruled out.

Example: Confounding

Drug X is being developed for Crohn's disease. Placebo, 10 mg, and 20 mg doses of the drug were administered in a clinical trial. Though no dose dependent effect was apparent, patients who achieved the highest serum concentration of the drug had markedly better outcome. One possible explanation for this outcome would be that the drug was effective but only the patients with the highest exposure to the drug achieved a therapeutic level and derived a benefit.

However, the alternate explanation is that better absorption may be correlated to better outcome – for example, in a patient with a gastrointestinal disease, less sick patients may absorb drug better, but they would have had better outcome regardless of whether they received the drug or not.

Mean, Peak, and Trough Dosing:

It is common to dose the drug to mean concentration, but in some cases efficacy or toxicity may be related to maximum or minimum concentration. For some other drugs, a drug holiday or drug free period (e.g., nitrates) may be important.

2.2.5.2 Pharmacodynamic-Based Dose

Sometimes pharmacokinetics alone is not a good predictor of clinical effect or toxicity. In such a case, a pharmacodynamic parameter must be used to dose the drug. For example, there may be a lag between dosing and effect or an interaction with another factor might make drug level alone not predictive of pharmacodynamic effect. In other cases, it may not be possible to measure the pharmacokinetics in a practical manner and pharmacodynamic measurements are required. Heparin is one example where pharmacodynamic parameter is used to adjust drug dose. With heparin, neither dose nor patient characteristics predict drug effects well, and international normalized ratio (INR) must be checked and used to adjust the drug dose for individual patients.

Pharmacodynamic endpoints are surrogate endpoints, and like other surrogate endpoints, they must be validated. Sometimes the validation is straightforward. For example 80% platelet aggregation inhibition for IIb/IIIa inhibitors is a well-validated surrogate that had been matched and validated against acute coronary events. In other cases, such as adhesion molecule inhibitors, the target inhibition range is not always straightforward. In that case, for example, it may not be clear whether the target level should be 90% saturation, 95% saturation, or something other value. It may not be clear also whether the dose should be sufficient to insure that the average plasma level is sufficient to achieve the target or it or the 10th percentile plasma level. In other words, the dose might need to be high enough to insure that the patients who have lower than the average response to a drug will still receive sufficient amounts of drug.

Just as for efficacy, sometimes pharmacodynamic parameters can be used to titrate the dose to minimize safety issues, such as fibrinogen depletion for thrombolytics, where extremely low levels of fibrinogen may portend an increased risk for bleeding. Fibrinogen levels can be followed, and the dose adjusted when the levels fall below acceptable levels.

2.2.5.3 Clinical Effect-Based Dose

In some cases, clinical response itself can guide dosing. For drugs like analgesics, this is eminently feasible and practical. Clinical effects that are immediately apparent, easy to monitor, and are reversible can be used to titrate dosing for individuals. However, the vast majority of clinical endpoints do not fulfill those requirements. Many are asymptomatic or hard to monitor, such as progression of atherosclerosis, or are irreversible such as stroke, or take a long time to manifest, such as osteoporosis. Irreversible events don't allow for titration, since once the event occurs, the titration no longer makes any sense. Also, in many cases the endpoint is the probability of an event, not an event itself, such as a coronary event risk.

In other cases, surrogate clinical endpoint can be used. Blood pressure and cholesterol levels are two examples. Sometimes a safety endpoint or a side effect endpoint can be used to titrate the dosing, such as LFT elevations or nausea.

2.2.2 What is the Target Dose?

Ultimately, the target dose is the dose that yields the best ratio of clinical efficacy and safety. In rare instances, such as with blood pressure or blood glucose levels, a surrogate endpoint is used to pick the dose, but in most cases, clinical endpoints are used.

Ideally, if the efficacy and the safety curves separate sufficiently, the minimally effective dose is the dose that should be selected. This is generally the dose that is at the beginning of the plateau in the standard dose curve. In some cases, the efficacy does not need to be so high and a lower dose can be selected.

If the efficacy and safety curves do not separate cleanly, then the choices are more difficult, and clinical judgment has to be exercised regarding where on the curve the appropriate dose lies, and what the appropriate trade-off of safety and efficacy is.

In selecting the quantity of drug, there are several considerations. First, it is not possible to test every potential dosing regimen. Second, there is a systematic bias toward underestimating the safety signal in small studies. Dose selection is generally an iterative process during drug development. The initial doses in Phase I are selected on the basis of animal data, and escalated carefully to assess initial safety. The Phase II doses are selected on the basis of safety information collected during Phase I, and in iterative clinical program, on basis of data generated in earlier Phase II studies. The Phase III doses are selected on the basis of the Phase II data.

2.2 Dosing Interval and Duration

2.2.1 Frequency

Small molecule drugs often have short half-lives. Biologics, which often have longer half-lives, tend to be doses much less frequently. Dosing regimen is usually dependent on the half-life of the drug, the therapeutic index, and the types of dose-dependent toxicities (and somewhat on speed of absorption). The dosing regimen can have a profound effect on efficacy and safety profile of the drug, and must be designed very carefully.

The exact methodology for calculating the dosing interval is beyond the scope of this book, and the pharmacokineticist should calculate dosages, but the clinical portion of the dosing decision involves the significance of the toxicities and the acceptability of the dosing interval.

For molecules with very short half-lives, such as epoprostanol (Flolan), or a very narrow therapeutic window, continuous IV dosing might be necessary.

2.2.2 Chronic *vs.* Intermittent Dosing

For acute diseases and diseases that flare and remit, short-term dosing or intermittent dosing may be appropriate. Antibiotics are archetypical short term drugs. For chronic diseases, though, chronic dosing is usually required. Antihypertensives, for example, are given indefinitely.

There are also some drugs that require a specific dosing interval, typically if tolerance develops. Nitrates is an example of a drug that requires a wean period.

Even more rarely, some biological systems respond only to cyclic patterns. For example, for gonadotropin releasing hormone, a steady, noncyclic pattern of administration antagonizes the effect of the natural cyclic endogenous hormone and results in downregulation of gonadotropin.

2.3 Initiation and Discontinuation

For most agents, initiation and discontinuation of therapy is straightforward, but there are several situations where special care must be exercised.

For some drugs, it is advisable to initiate therapy with a loading dose. If a drug has an inordinately long half-life compared to the speed of progression of the disease, this is prudent. If the drug has a different dose requirement for inducing remission than maintaining remission, a loading dose or induction dose(s) make sense. For a drug with severe symptomatic endpoint, such as pain, a loading dose might also be advisable, to relieve the symptoms as quickly as possible.

Also, a drug that tends to have side effects during a loading dose might require loading dose. For example, many drugs tend to cause QT prolongation, and *Torsades de Pointes* often occurs during loading. A rapid loading for several days in a hospital setting where the patient can be monitored may be preferable to loading over several weeks in an outpatient setting. Dofetilide, for example, is an antiarrhythmic drug that must be initiated in a hospital setting because of the risk of torsades, which tend to manifest itself during the 3 day loading period.

Some drugs have a first dose associated side effect, such as initial infusion reaction. This is not uncommon with biologics, particularly with antibody therapies. In those cases, consideration can be given to a lower dose at initiation of therapy (conditioning dose). Some drugs have toxicity that can be detected at low doses, where the side effect becomes greater at lower doses, such as methotrexate. In those cases, it is important to gradually increase the dose.

For drugs that exhibit rebound, discontinuation of the drug must be done carefully and sometime gradually. Benzodiazepine is an important example of such drug.

Some drugs have toxicities that can be detected early, that will influence continuation of the drug or continued escalation of the dose. Methotrexate is an example, as are statins. The adverse events tend to manifest themselves rather early because they occur frequently enough in patients who are susceptible to them that a defined length of monitoring at initiation of therapy can detect most of them.

Some drugs have narrow therapeutic index and/or the response to the drug is heterogeneous and must be titrated. Coumadin is an example. Initiation of such agents requires care. In some cases, there is a reasonably good predictive ability to guess the effect of the drug in advance, but the physiological or the clinical target has a range that must not be overshot. Blood glucose and blood pressure are two examples. Lowering those two parameters too much is detrimental. This is to be distinguished, for example, from clinical targets such as infections – there is no such thing as killing too many *M. tuberculosis*.

2.4 Route of Administration

IV administration is faster and assures more consistent drug delivery than oral administration. In instances where rapid onset of action is important, such as bacterial meningitis, IV administration is necessary.

In some cases, where bioavailability by oral route is not high enough, parenteral administration is the only possible route of administration.
The route of administration is dictated by oral bioavailability, need to control the exact dosing, site of action, etc. The choices include IV, oral, SC, IM, rectal, sublingual, pulmonary, vaginal, intranasal, topical, ophthalmic, etc.

However, oral administration is the more convenient and acceptable to the patient than parenteral administration. Formulating an oral drug, or designing a drug that is orally bioavailable can be difficult, since the dissolution, absorption, interaction with pH, food, etc. all must be optimized.

In some cases, the site of delivery is dictated by the site of disease – such as topical or rectal enemas for local disease.

2.5 Controlled Delivery

Controlled delivery includes slow-release drugs, controlled-release drugs (drugs that release with a certain profile), delivery at a certain part of the gut, implanted eluting devices (such as coated stents), implantable pumps, and so on.

With some drugs, such as angina drugs, where there is a biological pattern of the clinical phenomena, such as highest incidence in early morning, controlled delivery that delivers high dose at certain times may be very beneficial. Some biologics, such as GNRH, where the biological effect is more dependent on peak to trough cycling, the pattern of delivery may be very important.

Some drugs are designed to deliver locally to a certain part of the gut, such as mesalazine, so that the drug can be delivered specifically to one area. Other drugs are only active in the bladder.

3 Relationship between Dose and Response

3.1 Overview

The relationship between dose and response can take multiple forms. In most cases, both efficacy and toxicity responses are dose related. Higher the dose, worse or more frequent are the effects. The relationships are usually but not always linear, and in rare instances it can be U shaped.

In some cases, the response is not dose dependent, such as agranulocytosis.

It is important to recognize that clinical studies are usually powered only to detect frequent, dose-related toxicities. It is usually not possible to detect rare idiosyncratic effects without a large Phase IV type trial.

3.2 Special Circumstances and Interactions with Other Factors

As was mentioned, some toxicities do not manifest until enough physiological damage has occurred to overcome the natural reserve of the organ system. In an analogous manner, some toxicities do not become apparent until the patients are in a stressful situation or are challenged. For example, tumor necrosis factor inhibitors reactivate tuberculosis only in patients with pre-existing latent infections. Other examples would be hypokalemia (digitalis, antiarrhythmics) unmasking proarrhythmic toxicities, infection unmasking adrenal insufficiency (corticosteroids), etc.

The differences in metabolism among patients, and concomitant medications can cause tremendous differences in the toxicity profile, as can the concomitant food (empty stomach, grape juice, etc.), diet (green vegetables and coumadin), etc.

Some toxicities are intimately associated with the biological effect, and are merely extensions of the desired biological effect. Examples include intracranial hemorrhage with thrombolytics and infections with immunosuppressive agents. In such cases, it might be impossible to dissociate the toxicity from the therapeutic effect. Indeed, for biologic agents, the most common toxicities are exactly this type.

Some toxicities are associated with the target, for example, renal toxicity with calcineurin inhibitors or protein kinase c effects with protein kinase c inhibitors (because it is hard to target one protein kinase c and not others). In other words, some biological process are closely linked by molecule phylogeny or pathophysiology and it is difficult to dissociate them. Some enzymes and molecules serve multiple processes, such as ADP or potassium channels. That is why antidiabetic drugs such as sulfonylureas decrease myocyte preconditioning, since both pancreatic cells and myocyte depend on potassium channels for physiological function.

The chemical structures also cause side effects, such as side chains associated with particular side effects such as QT_c prolongation and hepatotoxicity.

It's important keeping mind that sometimes the metabolites can cause toxicity, as can excipients, contaminants, and host cell proteins.

3.3 Standard Model

In most cases, the starting point for dose selection strategy is a simplified model illustrated below. As with many other biological phenomena, the majority of drugs exhibit an S-shaped curve with respect to efficacy and toxicity. At low doses, the pharmacological effect is slight, and at a certain dose, the effect starts increasing at a rapid rate, and at a higher dose, the effect reaches a plateau and at doses higher than that there is no further increase in the pharmacological effect.

Most therapeutically useful drugs have the following efficacy and safety profile. The area where the curves exhibit hysteresis usually defines the therapeutically appropriate dose, unless high efficacy is required and some toxicity is tolerable, as is the case with some oncology drugs.

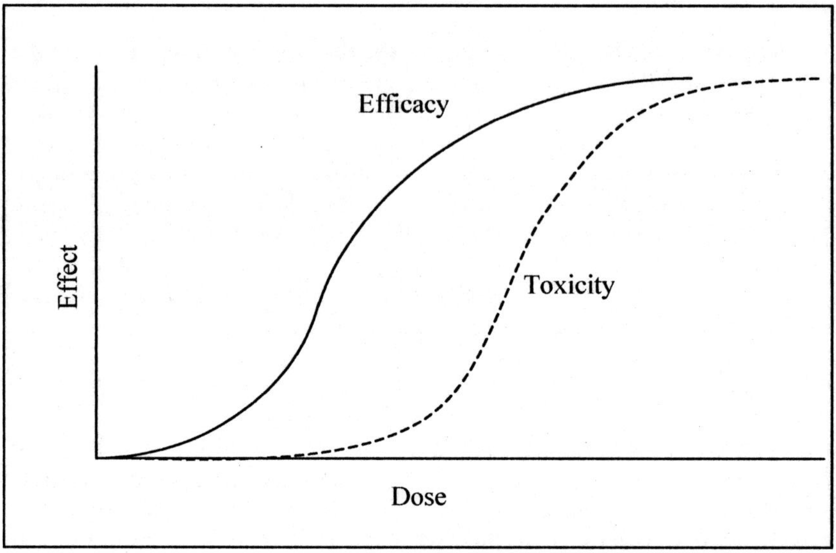

Obviously, wider the separation between the toxicity and the efficacy lines, better the therapeutic index. Not all drugs exhibit this pattern. If the separation is insufficient, or if they're reversed, the drug may not be useful as a therapeutic agent. An example of a drug that would not be acceptable is illustrated below. Of course, depending on the degree of unmet medical need, the type of efficacy, alternative available therapies, and the type of toxicity, the drug may or may not be of use.

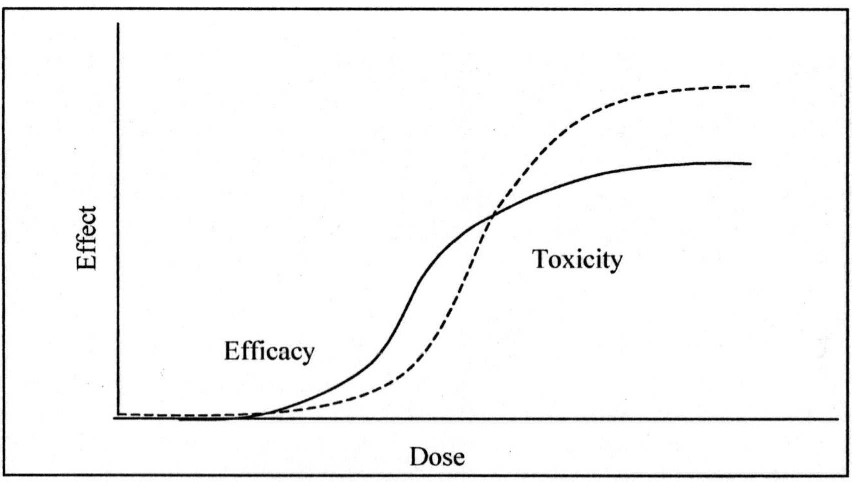

This model of efficacy and toxicity is obviously a simplification. Although useful as a starting point, this model has some major limitations, and relies on some important assumptions.

First of all, the model assumes that the efficacy and toxicity are dose-dependent. While this is usually true for efficacy, this may not be true for toxicity. For many drugs, particularly small molecules, the toxicity may be idiosyncratic. These include Stevens-Johnson syndrome, agranulocytosis, etc. where exposure to even a small amount of drug can cause the adverse reaction. This should be contrasted with cases where the risk of an event may be dose dependent but the manifestation of the risk is discrete, such as risk of cardiovascular event.

Importantly, different patients in a population have different response and toxicity curves. If the variability is high, then the curves may need to separate more widely than otherwise. For example, if the dose limiting toxicity of cardiotoxicity always occurs at 10 mg/kg dose, then the drug may be much more acceptable than a similar toxicity that occurs at average of 10 mg/kg of dose but with standard deviation of 5 mg/kg. With the first, it would be much safer to give a 9 mg/kg dose.

Depending on the drug, type of disease, and type of toxicities, the risk:benefit trade-off may be different. For example, if the drug is for hypertension, and the toxicity is fulminant liver failure, then the average toxicity curve is not helpful – what is important is the confidence interval that defines the 99.999% bottom of the toxicity curve (unless the toxicity is not dose dependent). This is because the risk tolerance for liver failure with an antihypertensive drug is very low. On the other hand, if the indication is acute myocardial infarction, then even intracranial hemorrhage toxicity may be acceptable at 1% rate.

The standard model also assumes that the dose response curve remains constant over time. This is not always the case. For some drugs, patients develop tolerance; while for others once a drug induces remission a lower dose may be sufficient to maintain remission. Also, the toxicity may be dependent not on current dose but on cumulative dose, such as with pulmonary fibrosis with amiodarone or cardiotoxicity with anthracyclins.

Monophasic or Multiphasic Response

Most drugs have a monophasic response – one plateau response curve. However, some have biphasic or multiphasic response. For example, a drug might have bacteriostatic concentration and bactericidal concentration.

U Shaped Curve

In rare instances, there is a U shaped curve. Typically this is a drug that has agonist-antagonist activity or in some cases drugs that depend on a gradient for effect.

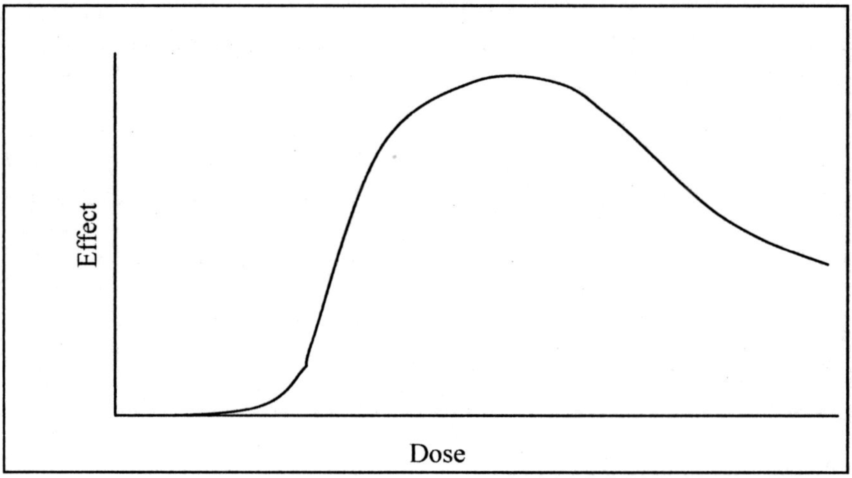

3.3 Dose-Response Safety Parameters

3.3.1 Overview

The most critical parameter in dose selection is safety. There are an infinite number of potential safety issues with drugs, but they can be classified into several conceptual categories, which are discussed below. It should be noted that many of these parameters are not specific to safety but rather can be considered to be general dose-response parameters.

3.3.2 Temporal Relationship to Drug Administration

The timing of the safety or efficacy signals relative to the administration of the drug has an important impact on the clinical trial design.

Some signals are acute and contemporaneous, and occur immediately upon drug administration. These include adverse reactions such as infusion reactions and nausea. These signals can often be detected with acute single dose studies. Some signals occur relatively acutely but with a slight delay after the drug has been absorbed had an opportunity to exert its effects within the body. Essentially, these are acute reactions but delayed by biodistribution. This is not uncommon and acute dosing studies are sufficient to detect these types of events as well.

The majority of safety signals are chronic and relatively contemporaneous. They occur during therapy, but after sufficient time has elapsed to unmask the effect. This can occur because of several different reasons. It can be because the effect takes time to manifest itself – for example, a drug that causes anemia by decreasing production of erythrocytes might not manifest its toxicity for several weeks. Or it can occur because the risk is low and it takes time before enough exposure has occurred to detect the signal. Unlike acute toxicities that tend to occur in almost everyone at risk as soon as the drug is introduced, chronic toxicity might occur only once every few months even in patients at risk. An example would be a drug that predisposes a patient to infections. The patient might need to be exposed to an infectious agent before the risk manifests itself.

Other signals occur on discontinuation of drug, such as rebound after beta-blocker withdrawal.

Temporal Relationship between Dose and Effect

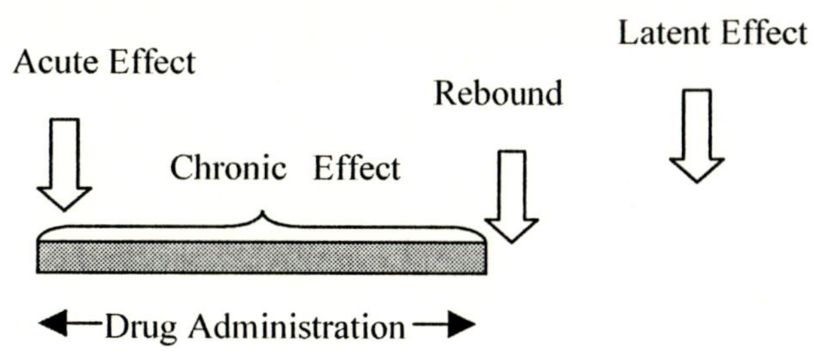

Other signals have a latency period, such as malignancies. They may not appear until years after drug administration. A classic example is psoralen long wave ultraviolet light (PUVA) therapy for psoriasis. Exposure to PUVA increases risk of cancer decades later, without short-term increase in malignancies. The risk manifests itself even if PUVA therapy is discontinued in the interim. Another is asbestos and mesothelioma. In these cases, the initial exposure might initiate or increase risk of a biological process that can take years to declare itself.

3.3.3 Relationship to Number of Doses and Amount of Cumulative Dose

As a first approximation, most drugs tend to have a continuous and constant risk of toxicity over time. That is, the risk of an adverse event over 6 months is half the risk of 12 months. The risk of an infection may be 1% per month regardless of whether the patient has been on the drug for one month or 20.

However, many drugs have a first dose effect, in that there is a side effect associated with first exposure that declines or disappears with re-administration. In other words, the risk declines over time.

Other drugs have increasing risk of toxicity with increase in cumulative dose. Examples mentioned earlier include cardiotoxicity with adriamycin and pulmonary fibrosis with amiodarone. Only after the patients have received a total dose exceeding a certain amount do the toxicities manifest. This is not uncommon because clinical manifestations of a drug may not be apparent until tissue damage has progressed enough that the body's reserve capacity has been used up. So for example, adriamycin causes myocyte damage even at low doses, but the heart can compensate for it in the initial stages. It is only when the reserve capacity has been used up that the clinical symptoms of congestive heart failure appear.

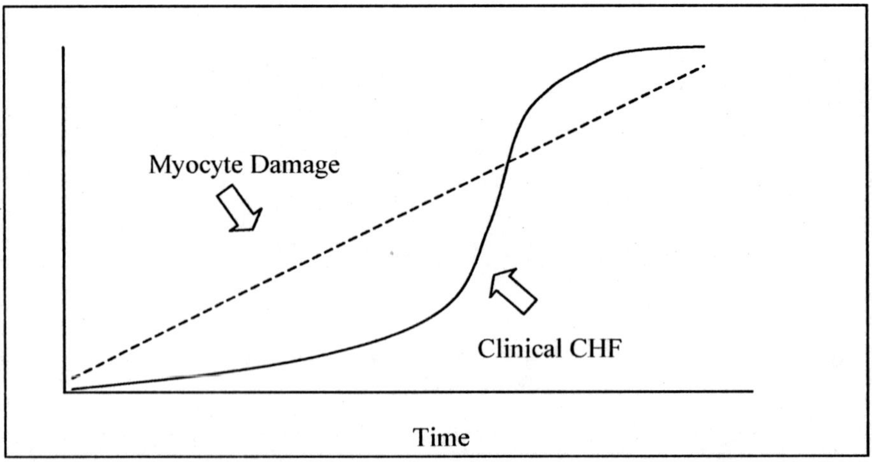

This should be distinguished from toxicities that have a constant rate over time but a low rate, such that only after enough patient have been studied for sufficient length of time do the rate for patients on drug separate statistically from the control patients.

There are some drugs with toxicities that manifest after long-term therapy because there is an exposure-response effect that is distinct from a cumulative dose effect. In other words, the risk of toxicity increases over time, but not necessarily in relation to dose. Doubling the dose doesn't decrease the time to toxicity by 50%, as is the case with dose-dependent toxicity. For exposure dependent toxicity, a drug holiday can ameliorate the risk.

Yet other effects appear only when the patient is retreated with the drug after a hiatus. Anaphylactic reactions can be of this type. The initial treatment induces an immune response, and a hiatus enhances the magnitude of immune response after a period without administration of the drug.

3.4 Efficacy Parameters

In determining the efficacy dose-response curve, it is important to define what elements of efficacy is being maximized. Efficacy can be described in many different ways, as listed below, and depending of the drug, one or more of the following parameters may be important. The target dose may be different for different endpoints, as may be the acceptable level of toxicity. For example, a drug that induces remission would be given for a short period of time, and acute toxicity is more important than cumulative toxicity, while a drug that is meant for long term maintenance, the opposite is true.

Elimination of symptoms or disease:

This includes acute endpoints such as resolution of pneumonia.

Decrease in time to resolution of symptom:

This includes endpoint such as length of oral herpes symptoms.

Prevention of symptoms or disease:

This includes chronic endpoints such as cardiovascular event or death.

Delay of symptoms or disease:

This includes endpoints that are likely to happen eventually, such as recurrence of atrial fibrillation or death.

Change in symptom:

This includes conditions such as blood pressure.

Speed in Onset of Action

This includes rapid relief of symptoms, such as time to improvement of headache. This is related to time to resolution of symptoms, but distinct, in that it captures the initiation of relief, as opposed to completion.

Persistence of Effect/Remission:

This refers to continuing effect even after discontinuation, though eventually the symptoms may return after a prolonged remission.

Lack of Tachyphlaxis:

This refers to ability to continue the drug with persistent effects.

Cure:

This refers to ability to resolve or prevent symptoms forever after treatment, such as after antibiotics therapy.

3.5 Convenience Parameters

Although safety and efficacy are well recognized as critical aspects of dose selection, convenience is often considered to be a secondary, optional aspect. This is a mistake. Here are the key convenience parameters, listed below.

Dosing Frequency:

Once or twice daily dosing are the preferred forms. Three times or more per day is difficult regimen for patients. Once a week dosing or less frequent has been shown to be acceptable, albeit sometimes with a need for reminder systems.

Weight-based *vs.* Flat Dosing:

Flat dosing is more convenient for patients and physicians and also reduces the possibility of calculation errors.

Dosing with Food *vs.* without Food *vs.* Either:

Drugs that can be given either on full or empty stomach, without altering dose, offer the most convenient dosing regimen.

Intravenous *vs.* Subcutaneous *vs.* Oral:

Oral doses are preferred significantly over parenteral forms. Subcutaneous administration is usually preferred over IV or IM, especially since it can be self administered at home.

Monitoring – Blood, Non-invasive:

Drugs that need monitoring, such as heparin, are less convenient to use. This is particularly true for self-administered drugs.

At-Home Dosing *vs.* Office *vs.* Hospital:

Usually, drugs that can be given at home, particularly via self administration, is more convenient than ones that can only be administered at clinic or hospital.

3.6 Confounding and Subpopulations

In assessing the effect of drug and doses, there are significant potential confounders. For example, some toxicities occur in a uniform fashion, while other toxicities occur only in a subgroup of patients. This occurs because of underling genotype (metabolic enzyme allotypes, for example), phenotype/concomitant diseases (renal insufficiency, for example), or exposure to environmental factors (smoking, sunlight exposure, etc.). For example, the 10% of the patients with the highest tumor burden might experience chills during the drug infusion.

There are many other factors that can affect the toxicity profile, including other interactions such as drug interactions, interactions with time of day the drug is given, season, diet, etc.

4 Response

4.1 What to Measure

As was discussed in an earlier chapter, endpoints can be classified into symptoms, signs, and laboratory tests. For purposes of dose exploration, these endpoints—sometimes called response variables—can be classified into several categories. Depending on the phase of the study, and depending on the goals of the study, one or more of these measures can be captured as endpoints.

One important aspect of dose selection is that many dose related responses, such as pharmacokinetic and pharmacodynamic, are not stochastic. There is enough reproducibility and low enough variability so that deterministic methods can be used with some pharmacokinetic and pharmacodynamic parameters. This is clearly different from the vast majority of endpoints used in clinical trials, and permits someone different types of analysis to be performed.

Clinical endpoints:

These include commonly used endpoints in late phase clinical trial such as signs, symptoms, quality of life, and adverse events.

Pharmacokinetics/Pharmacodynamics:

The pharmacokinetic measurements should include parent and metabolites, free and bound drug (bound to albumin, protein, antibody, ligand, etc.) Pharmacokinetic measurements are almost always performed on blood or serum, because it is difficult to measure the drug concentration at the site of action directly.

Pharmacodynamics refers to the biological activity of the drug *vs.* pharmacokinetics which refers to the amount of the drug. Pharmacodynamic effect can sometimes persist beyond pharmacokinetic levels, so it is often important to measure pharmacodynamic. Pharmacodynamic can also yield less variable measurements. Finally, it can also be easier to measure than pharmacokinetic in some instances, particularly when pharmacokinetic assays have not been well developed. For example, pharmacodynamic of a molecule that inhibits cell trafficking can be measured relatively easily, and more easily than it may be to develop an assay for the molecule itself.

Laboratory and surrogate endpoints:

These include endpoints such as ECG, pulmonary function tests, biomarkers (e.g., C reactive protein), and viral load. It also includes pseudoclinical endpoints such as blood pressure or diameter of coronary arteries that are not in and of themselves true clinic endpoints but can be meaningful markers of potential clinical sequelae.

Harbinger Signs:

Harbinger or sentinel signs are very important for rare adverse events. For example, nuisance bleeding with an anticoagulant such as gum bleeding may presage a more rare but more serious intracranial bleeding. Signs in patients under more physiologic stress is also an important item to examine. For example, patients receiving concomitant immunosuppressive agents along with the drug being tested might show signs of infection before those who don't, or the elderly might show signs of confusion before or at a lower dose than younger patients when they receive a drug.

Metabolites. Metabolism, and Alternate Forms:

Metabolites should be measured, especially if they may be active, have toxicity, or affect metabolism. Other measurements include alternate metabolites, endogenous ligands, fraction in a complex mixture (for example, different glycosylation forms for biologics), and enantiomer fractions. Heterogeneous mixture with several different half-lives can have complex elimination patterns.

Information about metabolism should also be collected. Principle routes of metabolism are liver and kidney, but metabolism in the gut and in the lungs can also occur. Information regarding liver metabolism should have been previously establish in vitro studies, usually using microsomes. This data should be confirmed and further investigated. The in vitro studies can yield information on whether a drug is metabolized by certain enzymes but does not yield information on relative contribution of liver metabolism *vs.* renal excretion or other routes of elimination.

If necessary, specific inhibitor studies can be performed with well-characterized P450 inhibitors such as ketoconazole (3A4) or quinidine (2D6). It is also necessary to investigate whether the drug can induce or inhibit metabolic enzymes, even the ones that do not metabolize the drug, because this can lead to drug-drug interactions.

Genetic Polymorphism:

Significant variation in genetic makeup that might affect metabolism or other factors in the action of the drug should be measured.

Substrates and Targets:

These are conditions are factors that the drug affects. For example, vitamin K would be the target for coumadin.

Effectors:

These are conditions or factors that must be present in order to potentiate the effects of the drug. One example would be complements for complement dependent cytotoxicity seen with certain antibodies.

Confounders:

These include serum albumin that can affect the free plasma level of a drug. It can also include concomitant medications that might influence the activity or metabolism of the drug. It could also include endogenous ligand if the drug is a competitive inhibitor or binder (beta blockers and catecholamines, Caastin and vascular endothelial growth factor).

There can also be chaperon effects. One example is with antibodies and biologics. For example, anti-vascular endothelial growth factor antibodies can prolong the half-life of vascular endothelial growth factor by binding to and sequestering vascular endothelial growth factor. Sometimes there can be sequestration or dilution of the drug by endogenous factors as well, such as when a patient has mutant form of a protein that dimerizes or trimerizes, and exogenous protein can be partially neutralized by dimerization or trimerization with the endogenous mutant protein.

Biomarkers:

These include items such as cytokine levels, levels of endogenous ligand, receptor saturation on cell surface, leukocyte counts, etc.

4.2 When and How Often to Measure

The goal of dose ranging studies is to characterize the relationship between the drug (or come parameter associated with the drug, such as pharmacokinetic) and endpoints. There are finite number of samples and timepoints one can measure, for both logistic and ethical reasons.

The frequency of measurements depends on the phase of the study, half-life of the drug, and therapeutic index. Early in the development of a drug, multiple frequent sampling might be necessary, and later in development, fewer. The goal is to capture enough data to understand peak concentration (C_{max}) shortly after administration of the drug, trough concentration prior to a repeat administration of a drug (C_{min}), absorption, half-life, interpatient variability, and a few other key parameters.

Population pharmacokinetics can be used in cases where frequent sampling is not possible and later in the program. Population pharmacokinetic relies on random or semirandom measurements, and mathematical modeling to estimate the pharmacokinetic curve.

Also, it's important to remember that although most toxicities occur relatively concurrent with the dosing, some effects will not manifest until some time later. An example is depletion of T-cells after administration of Amevive. It is therefore imperative to monitor the patients for sufficient length of time. The exact length of time depends on the expected mechanism of action, animal data, data seen in similar drugs of the class, half-life of the drug, etc.

It's also important that some toxicities will only manifest when the subjects are stressed. For example, an immunosuppressive agent may not show increase in infections unless the patients are exposed to pathogens. Or, the patients may not show diminished cardiac function unless they are placed on a treadmill. Obviously, it is not possible to stress the patients in many instances, but if it is possible to do so in a safe and ethical manner, this should be considered.

4.3 Reversibility of Endpoint

Some endpoints are real time and reversible, some aren't. Irreversible endpoints preclude certain types of common study designs, such as crossover or uptitration studies.

5 Designing Doses-Testing Trials

5.1 Goals

As was previous mentioned, dose–ranging studies have two goals: selection of the appropriate dose, and characterization of the drug's profile as it relates to different doses.

Dosing regimen is selected based on the risk-benefit profile, taking into account the severity of the disease being treated and alternative therapies that are available. The goal is to maximized efficacy while minimizing toxicity. More severe the disease and fewer the alternatives, higher will be the level of acceptable toxicity. One of the goals of early Phase (I and II) is to generate the data necessary to make a reasoned and data-based selection.

The investigation of dosing can be divided into several phases, each with different sets of challenges. Phase I studies define acute toxicities. Phase I study designs rely heavily on animal data and is a specialized area of clinical research. The goal is to escalate the dose carefully, to generate enough data about the drug, and to escalate to the maximally tolerated dose. In some cases, the maximally tolerated dose cannot be reached and the highest dose is a dose comfortably above the anticipated target dose.

Typically, the first in man studies begin as single ascending dose studies. Each patient typically receives a single dose of the drug, starting with a dose that is multiple orders of magnitude lower than the expected efficacious or expected toxic dose, and the dose is slowly increased. Each dose group is carefully monitored and the results of the dose group examined before the dose is escalated. The groups tend to be small, often with 6 patients or so. Placebo group is sometimes omitted from the early studies, although this is often unwise. Typically, the doses are escalated until a dose limiting toxicity is reached. Alternatively, if no dose limiting toxicity is seen, the doses are escalated until a dose that is expected to be the maximal dose required for efficacy is seen.

Multiple ascending doses are usually the next, and each patient group receives multiple dose of the drug, usually for a subchronic interval. Each dose group is assessed before the doses are escalated.

Phase II studies further investigate the dose to establish biological activity and the dose most likely to be useful. After single and multiple ascending doses, the drug typically proceeds into Phase II with 2-4 doses from the tested and tolerated doses. The goal of Phase II studies is to establish the dose(s) that will be advanced into Phase III. Subpopulation studies, such as studies in renal failure patients, are often performed during Phase II.

Phase III should be confirmatory, and the dose should already be selected in most cases. Phase III studies might include population pharmacokinetic studies to better characterize the effect of covariates such as age or sex on the variability of the pharmacokinetic parameters.

Phase IV studies often investigate additional dosing regimens or formulations.

A key issue in all phases is the quantity of data to collect, and the degree to which the drug profile should be characterized. It is impossible to collect complete data on all doses for a drug. Judicious choices must be made in deciding what regimens to test, and what extrapolations to draw from the data.

5.2 Key Factors in Dose Investigation

In order to determine the appropriate dose, data about the effect of the drug on the patients must be gathered. Because administering drug, particularly in an escalating dose fashion, to patients when the safety profile has not been fully characterized is a very risky proposition, and because the data has to be interpreted mathematically, the science of testing dosing regimens is a relatively complicated discipline. The key issues are listed below.

Starting Dose:

The first-in man studies start with an initial dose. This is generally based on the best available animal data, and the dose is generally calculated very conservatively, insure that the dose is going to be a no-effect dose. Typically, it is 1/25th to 1/100th of the no-effect dose seen in animals, adjusted for allometric scaling.

The paramount principle in designing the studies is protection of the patient. It is far more advisable to discontinue development of a good drug than to take risks that might cause injury to patients or volunteers. This principle has an important impact in the study design, since it necessitates non-parallel design, careful monitoring, etc. The goal is to place as few patients at risk to as minimal toxicities as possible.

Target Dose/Testing Range:

Ultimately, the dose chosen at the end of the program will be based on the clinical data from Phase III studies. However, a target dose must be selected at the beginning of the program, and the program must be designed to bracket this dose, because otherwise none of the tested doses may turn out to be a safe and effective dose. A common way of determining the target dose is to base it on animal work, with appropriate allometric scaling. Alternatively, it can be based on pathophysiology, such as 99% binding of the soluble hormone, or elimination of cancer marker such as alfa-fetal protein, etc.

One common mistake in selecting the target dose, however, is to ignore variability. For example, if it is known that 1 mg/kg of an antibody is sufficient to inhibit 99% of an integrin that's at mean expression levels, and average bioavailability if 50%, it may not be sufficient to administer 2 mg/kg if there is wide variability in either bioavailability of the drug or integrin expression levels. For example, if the standard deviation for bioavailability is 20%, and the standard deviation for the integrin expression is large, less than half of the patients may receive enough drug to inhibit 99% of the integrin.

Maximal Tolerated Dose:

For small molecules, the dose is usually escalated until signs of toxicity appear, which usually happens. For biologics, it is not uncommon to not have major toxicities with escalation until very high doses are reached. Maximally tolerated dose is the dose that is well-tolerated inmost patients – though for life-threatening indications, it could be the dose with some toxicities.

In general, with small molecules, it is ideal to establish a window of 5-10 fold safety margin for the dose that is ultimately taken into Phase III and marketed.

In cases where toxicity is not observed even at high doses, it is reasonable not to dose escalate beyond couple of logs beyond the expected effective dose/target dose. Also, the dose escalation should be stopped before reaching a dose that is 1/5th to 1/25th of no-toxicity dose in animals.

Minimally Effective Dose:

For many drugs, identifying the minimally effective dose is desirable to minimize toxicity. Finding a minimally effective dose is important particularly for small molecules, since small molecules tend to exhibit nontrivial safety issues at all doses. For small molecules, the minimally effective dose tends to the dose where the efficacy and safety curves diverge the most. Also, for a first-in-class drug for a disease without alternate therapies available, it might make sense to develop the drug as quickly as possible, so that it's available to patients as early as possible. For biologics, where the safety profile is often benign, finding the minimally effective dose may not be as critical.

The choice is between the optimal dose – finding the dose where the efficacy and safety curves diverge the most—and an acceptable dose, where the ratios of risk to benefit is acceptable.

In general, in order to determine the minimally effective dose, several doses must be characterized, with at least one dose being an ineffective dose, one dose being a plateau dose where there is not incremental benefit, and one dose being a toxic dose. With drugs with reversible toxicities—for example a drug that can cause torsades—it is not often prudent to push the dose to define the toxic dose.

Establishing a Safety Window:

Ideally, it is also ideal to establish a therapeutic window before proceeding with each phase of development and also for the marketed dose. For example, if the doses being marketed are 100 mg, having Phase II or 3 data with 200 mg showing lack of significant toxicity at the dose would be ideal, and is 100 mg and 200 mg are to be tested in Phase II, it would be ideal to have 400 mg dose tested in Phase I.

Speed of Escalation:

As was previously mentioned, dose escalation, particularly in Phase I, must be done with extreme caution.

Several different approaches to dose escalation can be taken, depending on the type of disease (oncology studies tend to escalate more rapidly), type of toxicity seen in animals, etc. For a drug with a potentially catastrophic toxicity, such as an anti-coagulant, gradual dose escalation is probably wise. One common escalation scheme is log or half log escalation. Alternate common approach is doubling of the dose with each increment. A Fibonacci schemes is sometimes used in oncology studies to reach therapeutic dose as quickly as possible.

Concomitant Medications:

Typically, early phase studies are conducted in patients without concomitant medications, to minimize confounding due to drug interactions. However, in later stage studies, it is often important to either conduct specific studies with commonly used concomitant medications or include such patients in the clinical studies.

Length of Subchronic Dosing:

The length of exposure in the clinical studies is largely dependent on the anticipated dosing in clinical practice. Other factors influencing it are the nature of the disease, anticipated onset of action, potential for rebound, potential for long term toxicity and potential for long term benefit.

In the early phase studies, such as multiple ascending doses in Phase I, 4-5 half-lives is typical, but if a drug has a very long half-life, then 10-14 days is common.

Length of Follow-Up:

The length of follow up after dosing also depends on factors mentioned in the above section. The minimum follow up, for safety is at least 4-5 half-life of the drug. For drugs with pharmacodynamic that is longer than pharmacokinetic, drugs that are sequestered or accumulate, and for drugs that exert a biological effect that is expected to last, the follow up will often need to be longer.

5.3 Testing Dose *vs.* Testing Pharmacokinetics/Pharmacodynamics

In cases where there is significant variability in bioavailability or metabolism, or in cases where the therapeutic window is narrow, it may be necessary to adjust the dose to target a certain plasma concentration or pharmacodynamic maker. For example, Xolair dose is designed to bring the IgE level down to below a certain threshold.

Commonly, the relationship between pharmacokinetic and clinical effect, or between pharmacodynamic endpoint and clinical effect is extrapolated on the basis of a conventional dose ranging study. In other words, the patients are given a predetermined dose, and those who happen to have the highest plasma levels are analyzed and compared to those who happen to achieve lower levels. This is prone to bias – for example, patients who have hepatic dysfunction might have the highest plasma levels, and might have the greatest toxicities not because of the plasma levels because of their underlying liver disease. Any time the study population is analyzed in subgroups defined by factors that arise during the course of the study, similar confounding factors are risks. For example, if it is found that patients who develop human anti-human antibody (HAHA) to a therapeutic drug such as remicade have less response to the drug than those who do not, it cannot be formally ruled out that the patients with more active immune systems happen to raise HAHA more easily and at the same time happen to have less response to remicade.

Alternately, the studies can target a certain dose level, and adjust the dose for each patient to reach that level (randomized, concentration-controlled trial). These are much more rigorous.

5.4 Characterizing Other Aspects of Dosing

As was previously mentioned, the issue of selecting the right dose is only one facet of dose testing. Dose characterization is also critical.

Special Populations:

Issues such as dose adjustment for special groups such as elderly patients, patients with hepatic or renal dysfunction, patients at higher risk of toxicities, etc. are important. In particular, the high risk group, if it is known that the drug will likely be used in the group, should be studied in carefully monitored studies, and before they are exposed to the drug in less controlled situation. For example, if one were developing an anticoagulant, with the expectation that the drug would be often used with IIb/IIIa inhibitors, then it would probably be prudent to study patients receiving a combination of the drugs in a controlled environment early in the program, rather than risk bleeding in a less controlled environment of a Phase II or IV. Pregnancies can also affect pharmacokinetic/pharmacodynamic.

Individual *vs.* Population Dose Response

It is absolutely critical to remember that the pharmacokinetic-clinical effect relationship can be different for patients and population if there is a large standard deviation. As shown below, even if as a population, therapeutic margin is large, the dose response on an individual patient basis may be steep, so titration for individual patient must be done more carefully in that case. For example, for a blood pressure medication, the average blood pressure for the group as a whole might decrease by 1 mmHg for every 1 mg increase in dose, but on an individual patient basis, the BP might drop by 5 mmHg for each 1 mg in dose. It's just that for each patient, the threshold where the blood pressure begins to respond is different. In such as case, it is important to examine the change in the endpoint rather than the absolute value against

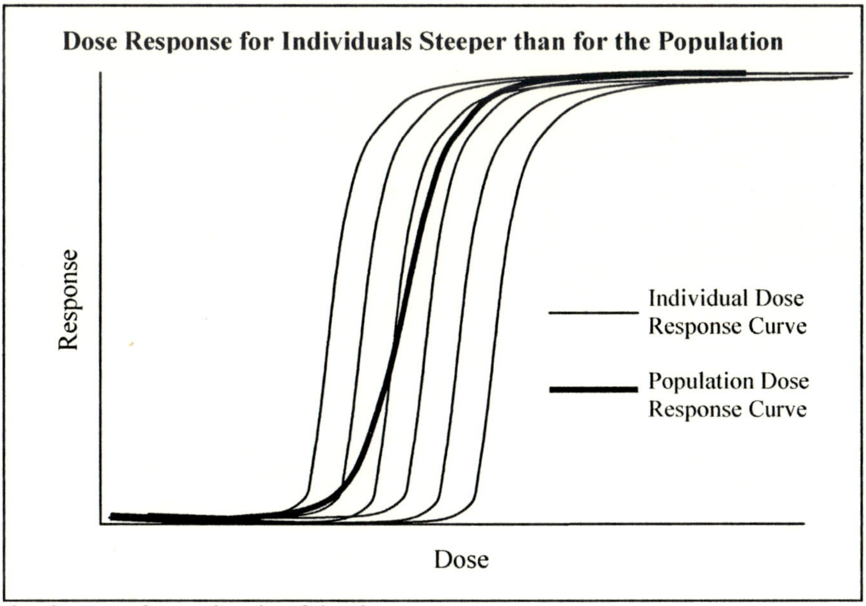

the dose or plasma levels of the drug.

5.5 Study Designs

Parallel *vs.* Titration Design:

For the most part, study design options for dose-testing studies are same as for other trials. However, because the trials are smaller, and usually generate data that will be re-tested in a later trial, designs that conserve the number of patients are often utilized for dose-testing trials. Two of the designs used frequently in dose-ranging trials are forced dose titration and optional dose titration.

There is an important bias in dose titration, because only the patients who don't respond get uptitrated. Because of regression to the mean, the higher doses will always have misleadingly high response rate when dose is uptitrated up.

Dose titrations are performed for one of two reasons. In one type of titration, it is necessary because the expectation is that in clinical practice the doses will be titrated. For example, blood pressure medications are typically titrated.

In a second type of titration, the goal is to re-use the patients in the clinical trial, either because they are difficult to recruit or because the interpatient variability is high. For example, a study of Gaucher's disease might specify dose titration because those patients are very difficult to recruit into the study. It is important to note that there is a bias in those types of studies because false positive responders will stop dose escalation while false negative will not. So the tendency will be to spuriously increase the safety and efficacy signals at lower doses if the test has low specificity, and to do the reverse if the disease tends to wax and wane. Alternatively, the most refractory patients may be the only ones who get titrated up, which would falsely lower the rate of response.

For some diseases, where there is variable response to the drug – for example, for peanut allergy patients in a challenge study – titration may not be appropriate, because the likelihood of having a response may be different for different drugs but each individual challenge may be positive or negative. Therefore, even if the risk of a response goes up, it may be difficult to detect or demonstrate it, because after the first event, patients cannot be rechallenged. It is then difficult to estimate the risk from one episode per patient.

Forced Titration (up or down):

In some dose-ranging studies, patients undergo titration in a lockstep fashion, with all patients receiving higher doses. In essence, this is a sequential non-parallel crossover design. This design was discussed in an earlier chapter.

The disadvantage of this design is that if the pharmacological effect is delayed, then the results could be confounded. It is not possible to determine whether the effect is due to higher dose or longer exposure.

Optional Titration:

In optional titration, each patient is titrated to an endpoint such as a clinical endpoint or a pharmacokinetic` endpoint. With this design, the critical bias discussed above is very common, that of the nonresponders being titrated to a higher dose. Sophisticated statistical deconvoluting may be required to analyze these types of studies.

Points for Consideration in Different Study Designs from the Exposure-Response Perspective (from FDA Guidance Document: Exposure-Response Relationships)	
Study Design	**Points to Consider in Study Design and Exposure-Response Analysis**
Crossover, fixed dose, dose response	• For immediate, acute, reversible responses • Provide both population mean and individual exposure-response information • Safety information obscured by time effects, tolerance, etc. • Treatment by period interactions and carryover effects are possible; dropouts are difficult to deal with • Changes in baseline-comparability between periods can be a problem
Parallel, fixed dose, dose response	• For long-term, chronic responses, or responses that are not quickly reversible • Provides only population mean, no individual dose response • Should have a relatively large number of subjects (1 dose per patient) • Gives good information on safety
Titration	• Provide population mean and individual exposure-response curves, if appropriately analyzed • Confounds time and dose effects, a particular problem for safety assessment
Concentration-controlled, fixed dose, parallel, or crossover	• Directly provides group concentration-response curves (and individual curves, if crossover) and handles intersubject variability in pharmacokinetics at the study design level rather than data analysis level • Requires real-time assay availability

6 Special Trials

6.1 Bioequivalence Trials

The standard requirements for showing equivalence, per FDA regulations, is a comparator head to head trial that demonstrates that the ratio of Cmax and AUC's 90% confidence intervals fall between 80% - 125%. These values are based on population values, rather than individual ratios. If there is a patient by drug interaction, there may be nonequivalence on the individual level, though, even if the two drugs are equivalent on population basis.

6.2 Special Populations

This is discussed in more detail in the following chapter, but if it is thought that the bioavailability or metabolism or excretion of the drug would be affected by concomitant disease, drug, or subpopulation characteristics, it may be necessary to conduct special studies in those populations. Whether to do so or not depends on a variety of facts.

For example, if preclinical or in-vitro models indicate that this may occur, it should be studied. For example, if p450 enzymes are affected, then it needs to be studied.

6.3 Hepatic Dysfunction Patients

Hepatic dysfunction should be tested if >20% of the metabolism is via the liver, or if the drug has low therapeutic index, or a large number of patients are anticipated to have hepatic dysfunction.

In general, at least 6 patients from Childs-Pughs Class A, B, and C should be studied. The control group should be the target patient population not normal volunteers, and should be age and gender matched. If P450 polymorphisms make a difference in the metabolism, then the patients should be matched for those as well, and larger number of patient may need to be studied. A smaller study may be sufficient in some cases where the concern regarding hepatic impairment is not as great.

A single dose study is often sufficient unless nonlinear pharmacokinetic or time-dependent pharmacokinetic is expected.

A population pharmacokinetic may be used in addition to or in rare cases in lieu of formal studies – but this would require careful pharmacokinetic analysis and screening of patients with hepatic dysfunction.

6.4 Renal Dysfunction Patients

Similarly, drugs that are excreted mostly by renal route, and/or have narrow therapeutic index should be assessed in renally impaired patients to determine whether a dose adjustment is necessary. Ideally, patients with the disease of interest should be compared to patients with mild (CrCl 50-80), moderate (30-50), and severe (<30) renal dysfunction and patients on dialysis. The variability of the pharmacokinetic and therapeutic window will determine the sample size, but the samples should be large enough to detect differences that would justify a reduced dosing schedule.

As with hepatic studies, a single dose study is sufficient if the pharmacokinetic is linear and not time-dependent.

Metabolites should be measured, not just parent drug, and free and bound drug should be measured.

In some instances, where the need for a full renal study is not clear, it may be sufficient to use population pharmacokinetic methods or initially test the severe patients only – with the idea that if the severe patients how no impairment, then less severe patients do not need to be evaluated.

6.5 Elderly Patients

In general, the pharmacokinetic profile in the elderly can be obtained by population pharmacokinetic or screening in the course of the program. I lieu of this, a formal pharmacokinetic study in the elderly can be performed. Most of the issues with the drug in elderly have been the result of altered pharmacokinetic, not pharmacodynamic, except in cases where the pharmacodynamic effect was due to conditions associated with age, such as decreased renal clearance or polypharmacy. If, however, a pharmacodynamic effect is expected – i.e., no difference in pharmacokinetic but a difference in clinical effect or pharmacodynamic effect, then those should be measured.

If the therapeutic window appears to be narrow, then the threshold for conducting the studies should be lower. If there is expected to be a large number of people with the condition – for example, diabetes in a patient population of congestive heart failure patients then the studies should be conducted. Most importantly, if the toxicity is severe, such as lactic acidosis, then the studies should be conducted.

In general, the studies examine the half-life and a dosing change recommendation is the goal. In some cases, it may be necessary to exclude certain patients from receiving the medication altogether.

This type of study is different from safety studies that are conducted in order to characterize the safety profile in a particularly vulnerable population where the drug levels do not change but the risk of toxicity does.

About the Author

Richard Chin is currently the Senior Vice President of Global Development at Elan Biopharmaceuticals, where he has worldwide responsibilities for Clinical Development, Regulatory, Biostatistics, Medical Affairs, Pharmacovigilence, CMC, and Quality groups. He has extensive experience in clinical research, and has overseen development and/or launches of multiple novel therapies including tenecteplase, efalizumab, alteplase (for catheter clearance), natalizumab, omalizumab, and ziconotide. Prior to Elan, Dr. Chin was at Genentech, where he oversaw approximately half of the drugs in the company's portfolio.

Dr. Chin holds an M.D. from Harvard Medical School. He trained at in internal medicine at Barnes Hospital. He also holds a law degree from Oxford University, where he studied under a Rhodes Scholarship. He was previously on the adjunct clinical faculty at Stanford University School of Medicine. Dr. Chin currently serves on the board of directors for Oxigene and on the scientific advisory board for Genmedica Therapeutics.

Printed in the United States
35844LVS00003B/7

9 780977 230228